Fill Up
to Slim Down

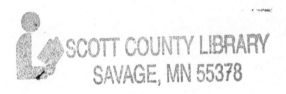

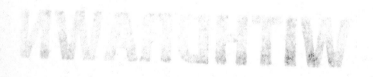

Also by Jyl Steinback

Supermarket Gourmet

Countertop Magician

Cook Once, Eat for a Week

Superfoods

The Busy Mom's Make It Quick Cookbook

The Fat Free Living Super Cookbook

The Fat Free Living Family Cookbook

Fat Free Living Cookbook from Around the World

Recipes for Fat Free Living Cookbook

Recipes for Fat Free Living Cookbook 2

Recipes for Fat Free Living 3: Desserts

Recipes for Fat Free Living 4: Breads

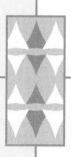

Fill Up
to Slim Down

THE DIET THAT LETS YOU EAT ALL THE
FOODS YOU LOVE AND STILL LOSE WEIGHT

Edward B. Diethrich, M.D.,
and
Jyl Steinback

AVERY
a member of Penguin Group (USA) Inc.
New York

AVERY

Published by the Penguin Group
Penguin Group (USA) Inc., 375 Hudson Street, New York, New York 10014, USA • Penguin Group
(Canada), 90 Eglinton Avenue East, Suite 700, Toronto, Ontario M4P 2Y3, Canada (a division of Pearson
Penguin Canada Inc.) • Penguin Books Ltd, 80 Strand, London WC2R 0RL, England • Penguin Ireland,
25 St Stephen's Green, Dublin 2, Ireland (a division of Penguin Books Ltd) • Penguin Group (Australia),
250 Camberwell Road, Camberwell, Victoria 3124, Australia (a division of Pearson Australia Group Pty
Ltd) • Penguin Books India Pvt Ltd, 11 Community Centre, Panchsheel Park, New Delhi–110 017,
India • Penguin Group (NZ), Cnr Airborne and Rosedale Roads, Albany, Auckland 1310, New Zealand
(a division of Pearson New Zealand Ltd) • Penguin Books (South Africa) (Pty) Ltd, 24 Sturdee Avenue,
Rosebank, Johannesburg 2196, South Africa
Penguin Books Ltd, Registered Offices: 80 Strand, London WC2R 0RL, England

First trade paperback edition 2005

The Library of Congress cataloged the hardcover edition as follows:

Diethrich, Edward B., date.
    Fill up to slim down : the diet that lets you eat all the foods you love and still lose weight/
Edward B. Diethrich and Jyl Steinback.
        p.   cm.
    Includes index.
    ISBN 1-58333-213-8
    1. Reducing diets—Recipes.   2. Appetite.   I. Steinback, Jyl.   II. Title.
    RM222.2.D565   2005   2004052911
    641.5'63—dc22
        ISBN 1-58333-248-0 (paperback edition)

Printed in the United States of America
10   9   8   7   6   5   4   3   2   1

BOOK DESIGN BY MEIGHAN CAVANAUGH

Acknowledgments

I would like to extend my gratitude to the thousands of patients over the years who have entrusted their cardiovascular care to the Arizona Heart Institute. My experience with them has contributed to the concepts and recommendations in this book.

—*Edward B. Diethrich, M.D.*

I want to thank these extraordinary people in my life who, like me, "Believed in Magic." They have helped me on this spectacular journey to helping the world become a healthier place. Thank you all from the bottom of my heart.

Gary, Jamie, and Scott, life doesn't get any better than these three people. Gary, thank you for your support in everything I do. Jamie, you are exquisite and I love you so very much. I am so grateful and blessed for having you as my daughter. Scott, you're amazing. I love you with all my heart. The three of you are truly a gift in my life and you fill my life with glory!

Mom and Dad, I love life. Thank you for giving me one that is so treasured with love, dreams, and believing in myself.

Jacie, Jeff, Diane, Alex, and Casey, I love you all from the bottom of my heart.

Grandma, Harlan, and Snooky, I love you!

Dr. Ted Diethrich, it has been a pleasure working with you, creating this superb book, and helping the world get just a little bit healthier. Finally, here's a healthy *lifestyle* for everyone to *live*! I have wanted to create this book with you for the past several years, for your vision of health and wellness matches mine. *Live it every day!* Thank you for all of your wonderful support and friendship and helping make weight loss a reality.

Mikki Eveloff, you are one of the most amazing and talented women I know. Thank you for sharing your friendship and tremendous gifts of creativity, perseverance, dedication, and a beautiful heart.

Debbie Kohl, we did it again, girl. You are remarkable and never give up. Thank you for your dear friendship and gentle strength to make it at the "wire" each and every time.

Coleen O'Shea, this is our fifth book together and I want to thank you for your encouragement and incredible support. I appreciate *all* that you do. Thank you, Coleen!

Barbara Alpert and Julia Vantine-Reichardt, you are both pleasures to work with and have been invaluable in orchestrating this book. Thank you so much for your creativity, research, and hard, nonstop work.

Kristen Jennings, you are a sweetheart and an awesome editor. Thank you for all of your wonderful guidance, positive energy, and expertise.

— *Jyl Steinback*

Contents

Recipes

Fill Up
to Slim Down

Introduction

Why Fill Up to Slim Down?

In the midst of a low-carb revolution, when sales of diet products are booming and shelves at bookstores and libraries are sagging under the weight of weight-loss books that feature everything from food combining reinvented by a former sitcom star to "get-tough" advice from a celebrated talk-show host, do we really need another diet book?

Simply, yes. Yes, because with everything that's been published and promoted—the diet books, the hundreds of low-carb products, the miracle supplements—more people are fatter than ever, and heart disease continues to kill or incapacitate more people than any other health concern. This means that what people are doing isn't working. That's no surprise, because most diets are viewed as temporary solutions, something you do until you reach your weight goal, and then go back to "normal life."

Unfortunately, normal life for many people describes an eating style that is unhealthy, a lifestyle that is sedentary, and a way of living that contributes to the development of medical concerns such as high blood pressure, diabetes, high cholesterol, cardiovascular disease, and stress-related illnesses that include ulcers, irritable bowel syndrome, debilitating anxiety disorders, and many more.

Part of the problem is the desire for a quick fix, a rapid reduction in the numbers on the scale and a drop in clothing sizes that can be instantly ego-satisfying. Look at all the TV and print ads extolling the latest miracle diet programs. These ads get results and these programs make a profit. But the majority of dieters in this country watch their hard-won lost pounds rebound back upward, again and again.

The result of these efforts is usually a slowed-down metabolism from the yo-yo dieting, a lowering of self-esteem, and a discouraging sense of failure and hopelessness. Some people blame themselves, while others blame their diets or their doctors. Many give up their attempts to lose weight and get healthier. But the rest start looking for the next new thing—the magic pill that will finally solve their health and weight woes.

But there is no magic pill, no perfect and effortless system that will solve this problem once and for all. That's the bad news. The good news is that it's possible to live and eat well for a lifetime, to reawaken your body's ability to heal itself, to renew your energy, rediscover a passion for life . . . in short, to fill up on the good stuff.

At Last! Feeling Full

The Fill Up to Slim Down program is designed to help you lose weight safely, effectively, and permanently—without feeling hungry or deprived. It emphasizes variety, moderation, and balance—without sacrificing flavor or favorite foods.

How? By using the scientific principle of *satiety*. Simply put, satiety is the tummy's signal that it's full. The Fill Up to Slim Down plan shows you how to sate your hunger on fewer calories by eating specific foods that can help you rein in your appetite. These foods contain specific nutrients known to help curb cravings—those unpredictable urges for a particular food like pizza, chocolate chip cookies, or ice cream. You'll learn more about satiety in chapter 1.

On the Fill Up to Slim Down program, you'll never feel as if you are on a diet. In fact, you'll be eating six times a day—three meals and three snacks! You'll even get to enjoy some of your favorite "bad" foods—every day, if you wish. The secret? We've devised a simple formula to help you plan your meals, which allows you to pick and choose what you wish to eat from lists of high-, medium-, and low-satiety foods.

At the end of this book, you'll find 120 recipes that can help you put the Fill Up to Slim Down plan into action. Far from dull, bland dishes that leave your tummy and taste buds wanting more, you'll find such favorites as Lasagna, Crusted Baked Salmon, and Chili Salsa Burgers. We've included breakfast ideas, soups, salads, main dishes, even desserts, all modified to make each serving more filling without adding extra calories.

But the Fill Up to Slim Down plan is about more than just food. It's also about moving your body regularly, to benefit your physical and emotional well-being. As moderate exercise helps burn off excess body fat, it delivers a couple of welcome bonuses. One, it tends to put the brakes on appetite. Two, exercise has been shown to reduce stress and boost self-esteem, which can help you stick to the plan. So as you select the best foods to satisfy *hunger,* your physiological need to eat, you'll exercise to help blunt *appetite,* which is the psychological desire to eat.

You'll also learn tips and tricks that can help you control stress, which can derail the most sincere attempts to eat right. Chronic stress tends to increase your levels of adrenaline (sometimes called the "flight or fright" hormone), as well as other stress hormones. Not only can these hormones make you more likely to overeat, they can also raise your blood pressure and cholesterol, which puts your heart in jeopardy.

In short, on the Fill Up to Slim Down plan, you'll eat more and crave less, move more and stress less, and within days you'll *weigh* less. More important, you'll keep off those pounds for good.

Shed the Weight, Save Your Heart

Of course, one of the best reasons to follow the Fill Up to Slim Down plan is to live a longer, healthier life. We promise that if you stick to the program, you will lose weight—up to two pounds a week!—as you reduce your risk of heart disease.

Doctors have long known about the link between heart disease and obesity, defined as an excessively high amount of body fat in relation to muscle (lean body mass). Body mass index (BMI)—a formula experts use to express the relationship of weight to height—is commonly used to determine overweight and obesity. A BMI of 25 to 29.9 suggests overweight, while a BMI of 30 or more indicates obesity.

Obese people have higher mortality rates from virtually all causes than normal-weight folks. In fact, according to one 2001 study, even being *overweight* increased the risk for developing major illnesses like heart disease, diabetes, stroke, and colon cancer.

Heart disease is the primary cause of death in obese people. Research has found that obesity hurts the heart in a variety of ways.

For example, there's no doubt that high blood pressure is the health problem most commonly linked to obesity, and that the more excess body fat you carry, the greater your risk. High blood pressure is defined by a systolic pressure (the top number of a blood-pressure reading) of more than 140 or a diastolic pressure (bottom number) of more than 90. Ideal adult blood pressure is 120/80 or lower. If you're carrying more weight than is healthy and you also have high blood pressure, you're risking heart attack, stroke, or enlargement of the left heart chamber, which is a major risk factor for heart failure.

Fortunately, it's now known that losing even a little bit of weight—as little as 5 to 10 percent of your total body weight!—can help reduce high blood pressure and the risk for heart failure. Plus, the Fill Up to Slim Down plan contains many of the foods recommended in the DASH diet (Dietary Approaches to Stopping Hypertension). This diet was created based on a large study of men and women that found that a diet reduced in total saturated fat and rich in fruits, vegetables, and low-fat dairy can significantly lower blood pressure. Because you'll be eating more of these foods and less processed and fatty fare, the Fill Up to Slim Down plan may well help lower your blood pressure.

Do you have high levels of triglycerides, an unhealthy type of blood fat, and low levels of "good" HDL cholesterol? Many overweight or obese folks do, and both are risk factors for heart disease. Again, the Fill Up to Slim Down plan's appealing blend of good-for-you carbohydrates from fruits, veggies, and whole grains and tummy-satisfying lean proteins and healthy fats can help you lower your total and "bad" LDL cholesterol. If you follow the exercise component of the plan (and of course you will!), you may also boost your HDL levels.

Eating and living the Fill Up to Slim Down way can also help save your arteries from damage. Research suggests that inflammation—the process by which the body responds to injury—may contribute to hardening of the arteries (atherosclerosis), in which fatty deposits build up in the lining of the arteries. The inflammatory response causes an increase in a substance called C-reactive protein (CRP), which is thought to heighten the risk of cardiovascular disease. In fact, studies have found that the risk for heart attack in people in the upper third of CRP levels is twice that of those whose CRP is in the lower third. By following the Fill Up to Slim Down plan, you'll be eating less of the fatty fare that tends to gunk up the arteries.

Not a bad deal: You'll slip into skinnier jeans while you also benefit the health of your heart. Best of all, you'll do it without a single minute of deprivation!

The Benefits of Satiety

If you've ever tried to quit smoking, you may know that within hours of stubbing out that last butt, health improves dramatically. For example, twenty minutes after quitting, the heart rate drops; in as little as two weeks after quitting, heart attack risk begins to drop.

Well, the benefits of switching over to the Fill Up to Slim Down way of eating can be almost as instantaneous. Here's what you can expect.

- Weight loss of ½ pound to 2 pounds a week
- Fewer cravings for the sugary, fatty foods that don't quell your hunger—and cause weight gain
- Reduced cholesterol and blood pressure
- Reduced risk of heart disease
- Reduced risk of other diseases, including diabetes and cancer
- More energy that lasts throughout the day
- Increased emotional well-being, self-confidence, and self-esteem

It's time to stop being hungry. It's time to seize the day, rebuild your confidence that change is possible, and reinvent your life in the best of health.

Hunger and Satiety: The Dynamic Duo

Remember that old Rolling Stones song that grumbled, "I can't get no satisfaction"? It's a perfect description of our country's epidemic of obesity. We eat and eat and eat, but apparently, we can't get full.

It may be that we can no longer distinguish between true hunger and appetite. They are vastly different, and the goal of the Fill Up to Slim Down program is to get you to understand these differences. When you do, you'll see why our program is so successful, and exactly how and what to eat to short-circuit the cravings and hunger pangs that may have plagued you on other weight-loss plans. You'll also understand why those high-fat, high-protein diets may not work well for you, especially if you're very overweight.

So forget the Rolling Stones' lament. Read on to discover why the Fill Up to Slim Down program will have you humming a different tune!

Hunger and Appetite:
One's from the Belly,
One's from the Brain

Many people use the words "hunger" and "appetite" interchangeably. For example, they may say "I'm hungry" just a few hours after they've eaten a meal.

But more often than not, what they're describing is *appetite,* the psychological desire to eat. Appetite is triggered by our senses, which are stimulated by seeing, smelling, or tasting food, or by our emotions, as when we recall a past pleasant experience with food. Appetite tends to be more specific, informing you that you want a particular food or foods—Mom's homemade chocolate-chip cookies, or a bag of crispy, crunchy chips. Even photographs of luscious brownies or a pizza oozing cheese can get your mouth watering!

By contrast, hunger is a physiological *need* for food. When you're hungry, you experience physical symptoms: your stomach rumbles, or you experience fatigue, lack of concentration, or grumpiness. These signals are your body's way of demanding that you provide it with nourishment. *Satiety* is the stomach's signal that its hunger has been quenched.

Here's the problem: Many people eat to satisfy their appetites, rather than their physical hunger. And as you'll come to understand, some foods satisfy hunger and promote satiety better than others.

For example, high-fat foods tend to please appetite, not hunger. It's easy to overeat high-fat foods like potato chips and double cheeseburgers and meat-lovers' pizzas. Why? Because they taste good, of course. But there's something more you need to know: High-fat foods *have a smaller satiety value than high-carbohydrate foods.* Simply stated, foods that are high in fat don't fill us up or sustain us throughout the day. As you'll see, our bodies are uniquely designed to tell us which foods will give us the most nutritional bang for the buck—and "turn off" our hunger switches.

THE "SATIETY HORMONES"

A number of hormones, or chemicals that interact with those hormones, have a powerful effect on satiety. They include:

Cholecystokinin (CCK): The body's natural satiety factor. Released by the intestine, CCK sends the message to your brain to stop eating because you are "full." Thus, CCK plays a powerful role in helping you naturally control your food intake and provides a kind of hormonal "willpower"—a helpful weapon in the battle against overeating.

Leptin: The "I'm-full" hormone. Named after the Greek word for "thin"—*leptos*—leptin stimulates nerve cells that release peptide hormones that help to control eating. It also decreases fat stores by raising metabolism. Leptin has been widely studied and has been shown to cause weight loss in test animals by reducing appetite and increasing metabolism. Recent studies are showing that while leptin can't cause weight loss, once the weight is lost some people regain their sensitivity to it and it begins to work again. So leptin may be of help in the long term in *keeping* weight off.

Amylin: This peptide hormone regulates food intake by providing feedback on appetite and satiety as well as the rate of food delivery from the stomach. Studies have shown that amylin slows the rate at which the stomach empties, thereby reducing food intake.

Why We Get Hungry—and How We Get Full

Hunger and satiety are controlled by the hypothalamus gland, the area of the brain that is responsible for metabolism, temperature regulation, sleep cycles, and, yes, hunger. The hypothalamus receives information from many areas of the body, including the stomach and intestines. When it comes to hunger and satiety, the hypothalamus can be compared to the gas gauge on your dashboard.

When the needle points to empty, the hypothalamus releases chemicals to the nerves of the stomach, which trigger hunger pangs. If you ignore these pangs—say, you work through lunch—the brain will become alarmed and produce a variety of chemicals designed to wipe out all other thoughts and desires but those for food.

When you finally eat, nerves in the stomach transmit different signals, and the hypothalamus registers your "tank" as being full. Then it releases other chemicals designed to get you to stop eating. (It takes about twenty minutes for your brain to get the "I'm full" signal to your stomach.) In several hours, when the stomach contracts and empties, you'll feel hungry once again.

Hopefully, you'll choose foods that promote *satiety,* the degree to which a food keeps hunger at bay. Thanks to a group of researchers in Australia, we now have a better idea of what these foods might be.

In 1995, Susanne Holt, Ph.D., of the University of Sydney, Australia, and her colleagues had a group of volunteers eat a 240-calorie portion of thirty-three specific foods, then rate their feelings of hunger every fifteen minutes over a two-hour period. During this period, the students could go to a buffet table and eat their fill, as the researchers watched.

White bread was given a baseline score of 100. Foods that scored higher than 100 were judged to be more satisfying than white bread; those under 100, less satisfying. Voilà—the satiety index (SI) was born. The take-home message: Foods with a higher SI suppress hunger longer.

The researchers found that foods that rank high on the SI have a number of qualities in common.

- High-SI foods such as baked potatoes, popcorn, and high-fiber cereals are bulky and high in fiber, which means that they require vigorous chewing and swallowing. These actions "massage" hunger pressure points in the body and signal fullness.
- High-SI foods such as oatmeal, apples, whole-grain pasta, and lentils help block absorption of fat and calories because they're high in fiber, which contains no calories, and because fiber speeds food out of the body.
- High-SI foods provide more energy from lean protein sources, including fish, beef, eggs, cheese, and beans.

The researchers' conclusion? Adopting a diet based on high-SI foods can help people trying to lose weight reduce the number of calories they consume *without* having to severely restrict their food intake or endure high levels of hunger between meals.

The satiety index is pictured below. Note: These foods are ranked *only* by the feeling of fullness a 240-calorie serving supplies, and the "servings" are not recommended as single servings—could anyone really eat four oranges at one sitting? However, the SI does make clear how much more you can eat of certain foods than others!

Food	Serving Size (each serving is equal to 240 calories)	Satiety Index Rating
Boiled potatoes	2 cups	323
Cod	8 ounces	225
Oatmeal	2 cups	209
Oranges	4 medium	202
Apples	3 medium	197
Wheat pasta	2½ oz, uncooked	188
Beef, top round	4 oz broiled	176
Baked beans	1 cup	168
Grapes	4 cups	162
Microwave popcorn	6 cups	154
Rye bread	4 slices	154
All-Bran with 1% milk	1 cup cereal + ½ cup milk	151
Poached eggs	3 large	150
Cheddar cheese	2 oz	146
Lentils	1 cup cooked	135
Brown rice	1 cup cooked	132
Water crackers	4 crackers	127
Chocolate chip cookies	2 large	120
Pasta	1 cup cooked	119

(continued)

Food	Serving Size (each serving is equal to 240 calories)	Satiety Index Rating
Bananas	2½ medium	118
Jellybeans	24 large	118
Special K with 1% milk	2 cups cereal + ½ cup milk	116
French fries	6 oz	116
Muesli	1 cup	100
White bread	4 slices	100
Vanilla ice cream	1 cup	96
Salted potato chips	25–30	91
Low-fat strawberry yogurt	1 cup	88
Salted roasted peanuts	½ oz	84
Mars bar	1 bar	70
Cinnamon doughnut	1 doughnut	68
Chocolate cake	1½ slices without icing	65
Croissant, bakery-style	1 croissant	47

 DOES DRINKING WATER REALLY FILL YOU UP?

Contrary to popular belief, drinking lots of water won't satisfy hunger pangs. But eating water-rich foods just might. In a study reported in the *American Journal of Clinical Nutrition,* researcher Barbara Rolls, Ph.D., of the Pennsylvania State University found that women who eat a bowl of chicken soup feel fuller than those who eat chicken casserole served with a glass of water, even though both meals contain exactly the same ingredients. Compared to those who ate the casserole, the soup eaters also tended to be less hungry at their next meal, and consumed fewer calories.

What's more, water can help you cut calories if you drink it in place of juices, sodas, and other beverages that contain added sugar. Like water, sugary beverages fail to trigger a sense of fullness, which means you can consume a lot of calories without satisfying your hunger.

But water isn't just your waistline's friend—it's a body-wide tonic. It regulates body temperature, keeps your metabolism revved, and helps your body eliminate all the high-fiber food you'll be enjoying on the Fill Up to Slim Down plan. There's even some evidence that being well hydrated may play a role in preventing cancer and heart disease.

The bottom line? Eat lots of water-rich foods to fill up your tummy and give your body the zero-calorie nutrient it needs to function at its peak. Drink at least eight 8-ounce glasses of water daily, including during exercise.

The Role of Fats and Carbohydrates

Believe it or not, your stomach gets the "satiety signal" from your brain. Satiety is regulated by the central nervous system via chemicals called neurotransmitters, which send messages to the brain. There are many kinds of neurotransmitters, and one in particular—called serotonin— has a significant role in the regulation of appetite. What's more, serotonin is activated by carbohydrates, especially complex carbohydrates.

This is how it works. Consuming complex carbohydrates increases levels of the amino acid tryptophan, a building block of serotonin. When tryptophan rises, so does serotonin. In fact, serotonin levels can rise within minutes of eating food high in complex carbs, such as half a whole-grain English muffin. Foods rich in *simple* carbohydrates, found in processed foods like boxed sweets and snacks, do *not* influence tryptophan levels as much.

What's more, complex carbohydrates have been shown to have a more powerful effect on feeling full than fat. Recent research suggests that routinely eating high-fat, processed foods overrides the brain's satiety signal. In other words, the more fat you eat, the more you want. The result? We keep eating when we're not truly hungry—and we gain weight. Additional research suggests that while dietary fat can diminish overeating in normal-weight people, overweight people don't seem to respond in the same way.

By contrast, researchers have found that fiber provides more bulk per calorie, helping your stomach feel fuller without your getting fatter. On the other hand, fats pack a lot of calories into a small space and leave you with a hungry feeling much sooner. The most satiating foods are high-fiber, complex carbohydrates that keep you feeling full for much longer periods of time than fats and proteins.

Also, foods rich in complex carbohydrates and fiber tend to have a low energy density. "Energy density" refers to the calories in a given amount of food. Foods with a high energy density contain a large number of calories in a relatively small amount of food, and often are high in fat or sugar.

Fresh vegetables, fruits, and whole grain carbohydrates such as pasta, baked potatoes, and brown rice have a low energy density—that is, they contain a small number of calories in a large amount of food. Foods with a low energy density consist of high amounts of water and fiber, so they take up more space in the stomach, take a relatively longer time to eat, and lead to a lower overall intake of calories. This promotes weight loss—without feeling hungry or deprived.

Foods rich in complex carbs also tend to fall lower on the Glycemic Index (GI), the measure of how quickly a particular food causes blood sugar to rise. Processed foods full of sugar and fat are high-GI foods, meaning they cause a rapid rise in blood sugar.

Chronically elevated blood sugar is not good for your health—or your waistline. A sharp, sudden rise in blood sugar can cause the pancreas to secrete large amounts of insulin, which can contribute to fat storage. High insulin levels can also raise blood pressure and triglycerides and lower "good" HDL cholesterol. This constellation of symptoms, called Syndrome X, sets the stage for heart disease.

FOUR FILL-YOU-UP TIPS

The philosophy behind the Fill Up to Slim Down program is simple: To feel full *and* feel healthy, choose bigger portions of low energy density foods while limiting those with a higher energy density. You'll find out the specifics in the next chapter, but here's a preview of ways to fill up without filling out.

Warm up to hot cereal. Oatmeal and other cooked cereals have one-fifth the calorie density of dried cereal. Hot cereal has 300 calories per pound; dried cereals pack in 1,400 to 2,000 calories per pound! Plus, hot cereal will keep you satiated into late morning, helping you avoid the midmorning munchies.

Pop to it. Need a snack? You can't do better than popcorn. Six cups of "light" microwave popcorn—hold the butter flavor, please—will satisfy you more than two small cookies.

Go green before each meal. Scientists at the Pennsylvania State University recently found that volunteers who ate a large salad before their main course ate fewer calories overall than those who didn't eat a salad first. (Watch the high-fat dressings, though—use a low-fat, low-calorie dressing instead.)

Pick lean protein over fattier meats. Extra-hungry at dinner? Eight ounces of broiled fish will fill your tummy better than a 4½-ounce steak.

Handling Hunger Better

The goal of the Fill Up to Slim Down program is to get you to see the importance of satisfying *hunger,* rather than appetite. You can do that by primarily choosing foods with a low-energy density and a low glycemic index rating. The Glycemic Index (GI) is a ranking system for carbohydrates based on how quickly they raise blood glucose and blood sugar. Plenty of tasty foods fit the bill, including low-fat cheeses and dairy, eggs, lean meats and fish, sweet fruits, tender-crisp fresh vegetables, and dense, nutty-tasting whole-grain breads, cereals, and pastas. These foods satisfy your hunger with fewer calories, even though you're eating "more." So cravings will fade, hunger pangs will go away, and you'll leave the table feeling full—neither stuffed nor starving.

We'll get into the particulars of the Fill Up to Slim Down program in the next chapter. But here's a little hint of how it works. Let's turn our attention to breakfast, a meal that is frequently rushed or even skipped altogether.

Breakfast Scenario 1: Just before you fly out the door, you gulp a glass of orange juice and grab a couple of cookies "to tide you over" until lunch. But by the time you reach your desk, you're hungry again, so you devour half a jelly doughnut. At 10 A.M., your stomach's rumbling again, so you filch a few mini candy bars from the jar on a colleague's desk. By the time lunchtime rolls around . . . look out! You're ready to eat anything that isn't nailed down.

Breakfast Scenario 2: You're still flying out the door, but this time you grab a no-peel piece of fruit (an apple, pear, or peach) and munch while you toast a whole-wheat English muffin. Topped with a slice of low-fat cheese, you've got a meal that will stick with you. Why? Because unlike the juice, the whole fruit contains bulk and fiber that takes up belly space. The whole-wheat English muffin with cheese delivers more of a fill-you-up mix of complex carbs and lean protein. You'll likely feel hungry at midmorning, which is natural—the body is designed to eat every three hours or so. So go ahead, have a snack—just choose a satisfying food in a sensible portion size.

2 Eat to Fill Up!

When you design your meals around the concept of satiety, you won't suffer what so many dieters complain about: hunger! The foods on the Fill Up to Slim Down program help you feel full *naturally,* for longer periods of time, so you're less likely to succumb to unplanned and unhealthy eating. And because you'll eat every few hours, you won't experience the cravings and ravenous hunger that low blood sugar can trigger.

Just as important, you'll eat foods that you love—sweet and juicy fruits, whole-grain breads and pastas, sweet potatoes, rice. Yes, we're talking about carbohydrates.

In recent years, carbohydrates have been the victim of a lot of bad press, and more than a few low-carb diet plans have found their way onto the bestseller lists. But what isn't said enough is that it's not "carbohydrates" that cause weight gain: It's the simple carbs like white flour, white sugar, soda, and other sweet-and-fatty foods that have made America the fattest nation on earth. So it simply isn't accurate to say that a "low-carb" diet is better for you. It's a diet that's low in processed simple carbohydrates that truly benefits your health and your waistline.

What's more, although proteins are essential, most Americans already eat more protein than their bodies need. Excess dietary protein can lead to increased health risks. Plus, a calorie is a calorie is a calorie. So if you eat too many calories from fat, they'll go straight to your hips—just like excess calories from carbohydrates will.

Why Low-Fat, "Smart-Carb" Is the Way to Go

So despite what the low-carb gurus say, it's undeniable that carbohydrates provide the body with its main source of energy. Here's even more ammunition for low-fat, good-carb eating:

1. Fat has 9 calories per gram, whereas carbohydrates and protein have 4 calories per gram. That means it's much easier to eat fewer calories when you limit dietary fat.

2. Studies show the body is less efficient at converting carbohydrates into body fat than fat into body fat. It takes your body only 2.5 calories to store 100 fat calories of body fat. But it must spend 23 calories to convert 100 calories of dietary carbs or protein into body fat.

3. Complex carbohydrates are high in fiber, which slows down the absorption of foods, so that you feel comfortably full for extended periods of time on a modest caloric intake.

4. A low-fat "healthy-carb" diet contains different kinds of fiber, which benefit your health in different ways. Insoluble fibers reduce the risk of serious conditions like diverticulosis and colon cancer, as well as common ones like constipation and

hemorrhoids. Soluble fibers help remove cholesterol from the body. They also slow the absorption of carbohydrates into your blood, so your blood-sugar levels remain steady. As it turns out, this is important for sustained weight loss.

But that's not all. Healthy carbohydrates contain phytochemicals—naturally occurring substances in plants that have been found to lessen the risk of diabetes, heart, and a host of other killer diseases. Eliminate most of the carbohydrates from your diet, and you eliminate the foods that may be your most potent allies in the fight against disease.

The good news is, you don't have to give them up to lose weight and keep it off.

 MORE EVIDENCE THAT LOW-CARB CAN'T CUT IT

1. In the most comprehensive study of long-lasting weight loss ever conducted, called the National Weight Control Registry, scientists studied more than 4,500 people who lost, on average, sixty-six pounds and kept it off for six years. The vast majority followed a diet low in fat and high in natural, fiber-rich carbohydrates like fruits and vegetables. Less than 1 percent followed a high-fat, high-protein diet.

2. According to a study conducted by the Veterans Administration Medical Center in Minneapolis, people who ate high-fiber cereal for breakfast consumed 150 to 200 fewer calories at lunch than those who'd started their day with a low-fiber choice.

3. Whole-grain bread's chewy fiber makes it three times as filling as an airy croissant, and 57 percent more satisfying than white bread. Bulk up a sandwich with lettuce, tomatoes, and sprouts, rather than cheese and meat.

The Fill-You-Up Food Groups

Eating the right balance of foods from the major food groups is the foundation of day-to-day well-being. When you eat the Fill Up way, most of your daily menu is made up of complex carbohydrates, followed by lean proteins and low-fat dairy products. You stand to reap two significant benefits: weight loss and a reduction of your long-term risk of disease. Let's take a closer look at what you'll be enjoying.

VEGETABLES

In this category, as well as the fruit category below, you'll be eating all the colors of the rainbow. Research shows that the brighter the hue of the veggie or fruit, the more health-enhancing nutrients it contains. In this category, feel free to exceed the recommended servings to feel fully satisfied. We recommend that you opt for fresh veggies as much as possible. If you can't, opt for frozen, which contain just as many nutrients.

FULFILLING SERVING SIZES: VEGETABLES

The number of recommended servings can be increased as you choose. Aim for a variety of textures and colors—choose crunchy as well as soft vegetables, those with higher and lower water content. *What's a Serving?* Half a cup of cooked vegetables; one to two cups of salad greens.

50+ adults:	3		
Women:	3	Active women:	4
Men:	4	Active men:	5
Teen girls:	4	Teen boys:	5
Children (ages 6 to 12):	4	Children (ages 2 to 6):	3

FRUITS

Being naturally sweet, fruit makes a perfect dessert or between-meal snack. Whole fresh fruit provides lots of healthy fiber and an abundance of vitamin C and other nutrients, while dried fruit is a concentrated source of nutrients and fiber. (Go easy on dried fruit, however—it is also a concentrated source of calories.)

Choose your fruit servings from the best seasonal fresh fruit. Frozen fruit and berries are fine, too, as is canned fruit. Using canned peaches in light syrup or juice is the best choice, because they are lower in calories and have less sugar. There's a wide variety of fruit to choose from, from old favorites like apples and oranges (which figure high on the SI, as you recall) to exotic fruits like kiwi and pomegranates. Try them all!

FULFILLING SERVING SIZES: FRUIT

Aim for a variety of colors as well as of fruit. Choose at least one citrus fruit (orange, grapefruit, tangerine) per day if possible. For greater satiety, eat whole fruit instead of drinking juice. *What's a Serving?* One whole fruit about the size of your fist; one cup of berries; half a cup of juice; one three-inch slice of melon; one-third to half a medium cantaloupe.

50+ adults:	2		
Women:	2	Active women:	3
Men:	3	Active men:	4
Teen girls:	3	Teen boys:	4
Children (ages 6 to 12):	3	Children (ages 2 to 6):	2

WHOLE GRAINS

These healthy carbohydrates take longer to digest and provide excellent fuel for the demands of your daily life (and exercise). Your best choices include brown rice, bulgur, oats (oatmeal, oat flour), pearl barley, and whole-grain cereals. These foods are high in fiber, provide lots of important nutrients, and offer plenty of options to plain meals and snacks.

FULFILLING SERVING SIZES: WHOLE GRAINS

Recommended servings vary greatly based on age and activity level. For example, if you're an active woman over fifty, you're likely to require more than six servings per day. If you're a sedentary woman, start with six servings and increase them as you raise your activity level. *What's a Serving?* One slice of whole-grain bread; one cup cooked or cold cereal; two ounces dry beans; a quarter cup barley or other grain; three cups popped popcorn; half a cup brown rice; half a cup pasta.

50+ adults:	6		
Women:	6	Active women:	9
Men:	9	Active men:	11
Teen girls:	9	Teen boys:	11
Children (ages 6 to 12):	9	Children (ages 2 to 6):	6

DAIRY PRODUCTS

Low-fat or non-fat dairy products like cheese, milk, and yogurt have all the calcium but little or none of the fat found in the full-fat versions— and they offer protein and bone-protective calcium, too. What's more, consuming several servings of low-fat dairy a day may help melt away those extra pounds. Previous studies have shown that calcium can boost weight loss by increasing fat breakdown in fat cells.

FULFILLING SERVING SIZES: DAIRY PRODUCTS

For all age groups, the recommendations are the same: select two to three servings per day. *What's a Serving?* One ounce of low-fat hard cheese; half a cup low-fat cottage cheese or ricotta; one cup low-fat milk; six to eight ounces low-fat or fat-free yogurt. If you don't eat dairy products, another source of calcium is raw tofu (1 cake) or collard or turnip greens, which are rich in calcium.

PROTEINS

While protein is essential to all aspects of the body's development, growth, and maintenance, you don't need much. In fact, only 13 to 20 percent of your daily calories should come from protein, and the typical American consumes far more than that, particularly if they're following a low-carbohydrate diet.

Meat, poultry, fish, dried beans, lentils, and eggs are good sources of lean protein, as well as the B vitamins, iron, and zinc. Cold water fish (salmon, tuna, herring, and sardines) contain omega-3 fatty acids—"good fats" that lower cholesterol and decrease the risk of heart disease.

FULFILLING SERVING SIZES: PROTEINS

Research shows that Americans eat far more protein than they need, especially in the form of meat. Experts suggest filling your plate with vegetables and grains, and "garnishing" the meal with meat. *What's a Serving?* Three

(continued)

ounces of cooked meat, fish, poultry; half a cup tofu or legumes; one egg; two tablespoons peanut or other nut butters; one-third cup nuts.

50+ adults:	5 ounces		
Women:	5 ounces	Active women:	6 ounces
Men:	6 ounces	Active men:	7 ounces
Teen girls:	6 ounces	Teen boys:	7 ounces
Children (ages 6 to 12):	6 ounces	Children (ages 2 to 6):	5 ounces

What About Fat?

Believe it or not, some fats are actually good for you—if you consume them in the proper amounts. These "healthy fats" are the unsaturated fats in products derived from plant sources, such as vegetable oils, nuts, and seeds. *Polyunsaturated fats* are found in high concentrations in safflower, sunflower, corn, and soybean oils, while *monounsaturated fats* are found in olive, peanut, and canola oils as well as nuts, olives, and avocados. In studies in which polyunsaturated and monounsaturated fats were eaten in place of saturated fat, LDL cholesterol decreased and HDL cholesterol increased.

Artery-clogging saturated fats are found in red meat and full-fat dairy products, as well as trans fats (also called hydrogenated or partially hydrogenated oils). These fats are formed when polyunsaturated oils are changed into saturated fats via the hydrogenation process—when corn oil is changed into margarine, for example. Trans fats may raise bad cholesterol even more than saturated fats. A large national study called the Nurses' Health Study found that replacing just 30 calories of carbohydrates every day with 30 calories of trans fats nearly doubled the risk for heart disease. Saturated fats increased risk as well, but not nearly as much.

All age groups should limit intake of these unhealthy fats to no more than 20 to 30 percent of total calories per day. Limit saturated fats to 7 percent of daily calories or less, and keep dietary cholesterol to 200 milligrams per day or less. (Parents, please note: Do not put children under age two on a fat-restricted diet. They need fat and cholesterol for proper growth and development of the brain, bones, and muscles.) To limit your intake of bad fats, see chapter 9.

FIBER: A DIETER'S BEST BUDDY

That eating a high-fiber diet benefits your health isn't news. But did you also know . . .

1. that dietary fiber contains no calories because the body can't absorb it?
2. that fiber's ability to absorb water makes you feel "full"?
3. that fiber-rich foods require more chewing, so you're just not able to eat a large number of calories in a short amount of time?

It's no coincidence that eight of the top ten most satisfying foods on the Satiety Index are high in fiber. That's right—if you're trying to shed pounds, fiber is your best friend! Here's a list of the best choices for getting all the benefits of high-fiber eating:

1. Dried beans, peas, and other legumes
2. Bran cereals (best bets: Bran Buds and All-Bran; 100% Bran, Raisin Bran, Most, and Cracklin' Oat Bran are also excellent sources.)
3. Fresh or frozen lima beans, both Fordhook and baby limas
4. Fresh or frozen green peas
5. Dried fruit, especially figs, apricots, and dates
6. Raspberries, blackberries, and strawberries

(continued)

7. Sweet corn, whether on the cob or cut off as kernels
8. Whole-wheat and other whole-grain cereal products (includes grains and grain products made from rye, oats, buckwheat, and stone-ground cornmeal)
9. Broccoli
10. Baked potato with the skin (the skin, when crisp, is the best part for fiber)
11. Green snap beans, pole beans, and broad beans
12. Plums, pears, and apples (eat the skin for extra fiber)
13. Raisins and prunes
14. Greens (spinach, beet greens, kale, collards, Swiss chard, turnip greens)
15. Nuts, especially almonds, Brazil nuts, and walnuts (pay particular attention to portion size; they're high in calories and fat)
16. Cherries
17. Bananas
18. Carrots
19. Coconut (dried or fresh, but both are high in fat)
20. Brussels sprouts

The Fill Up to Slim Down Plan

When you're trying to give your diet a healthy makeover, the thirty-three foods on the Satiety Index are a great place to start. But there are a lot of other great foods that can provide high satiety and promote weight loss. For the Fill Up to Slim Down program, we have greatly expanded the SI to include a wide variety of healthful foods that can provide high satiety and promote weight loss. There is even room for occasional low SI foods like desserts as a special treat.

Because many people are unwilling or unable to count servings of each food group, we wanted to make the Fill Up to Slim Down way of eating easy to remember and simple to use. The results: A "formula" with which you can customize your own meals and menus, using the lists of high-satiety (HS) foods and medium-satiety (MS) foods shown below. We call it the Fill Up Formula. You don't have to count fat or carbohydrate grams—you don't even have to count calories!

You'll enjoy three meals and three snacks a day. Simply consult the food lists shown below and create a meal based on the lists and the formula that follows.

Of course, you must pay attention to portions—that is, *how much* of any one food you're eating—as well as serving size, which is how many portions you can have per day, based on such factors as age, height, and activity level. Watching portions and serving size is a critical part of the success of this or any healthy eating plan. Remember, however, that you can exceed the recommended serving sizes in order to feel full. (Starchier veggies like corn and potatoes are more filling, so you will not require as much.)

One *meal*—breakfast, lunch, or dinner—is comprised of two servings of HS foods (one of which must be a fruit or veggie) plus one serving of MS food.

One *snack* is comprised of one to two servings of HS or MS foods, one of which must be a fruit or veggie.

You may also enjoy two servings of a low-satiety (LS) food per week, if you choose to. Remember, you'll lose weight more quickly if you try to avoid these foods altogether. If you do choose to have them, be conscious of portion size. One scoop of ice cream, for example, is the size of a tennis ball.

How does the Fill Up Formula work in real life? Well, for a woman, breakfast might be one egg and one piece of whole-grain toast (two servings of HS foods), coupled with a half cup of berries (one serving of MS food).

Lunch might be salad greens topped with three ounces of tuna (two servings of HS foods), and one apple or pear (one serving of MS food).

Dinner might be one hamburger on a whole-grain bun (two servings of HS foods), with a half cup of broccoli (one serving of MS food).

Your first snack might be one serving of cottage cheese with one peach (one serving of HS food plus one serving of MS food), while snack

2 might be one serving of air-popped popcorn with broccoli and fat-free dip. And you've still got one more snack to go!

See how easy it is? Create your meals and snacks from the lists below, which categorize foods according to their ability to satisfy hunger. A combination of the foods from this list eaten throughout the day will be the most satisfying. Using the recipes provided in this book will enhance the variety in your meal plan.

High Satiety

Lean proteins
Beans, black
Beans, garbanzo
Beans, green
Beans, kidney
Beans, navy
Beans, pinto
Beans, soy (edamame)
Beef, ground, lean
Beef, lean cuts
Cheese, any kind, low-fat or fat-free
Cheese, cottage, 1% or 2% milk fat
Cheese, soy
Chicken, ground
Chicken breast, prepared without fat, skin removed
Deli meats, lean (lean roast beef, ham, chicken breast, turkey breast)
Eggs, prepared without fat
Eggs, whites only
Egg substitutes
Fish and shellfish, baked, grilled, or broiled, prepared without fat
Lentils
Milk, low-fat or skim
Nuts, all varieties
Pork, lean cuts

Tofu, tempeh, cooked soybeans, and other soy proteins
Turkey, ground
Turkey breast, prepared without fat, skin removed
Veal
Yogurt, plain

Fiber-rich vegetables
Artichokes
Arugula
Asparagus
Beans, wax
Bok choy
Broccoli
Broccoli rabe
Brussels sprouts
Cabbage, green or red
Carrots
Cauliflower
Celery
Collards
Corn on the cob
Eggplant
Lettuce, all varieties
Mustard greens
Parsnips
Peas
Peppers, all colors
Potatoes, sweet
Potatoes, white, baked
Pumpkin
Spinach
Squash, summer (zucchini, yellow squash)
Squash, winter (butternut, acorn)
Swiss chard

Turnips
Yams

Fiber-rich fruits
Apples
Oranges
Pears
Strawberries, blueberries, raspberries, blackberries

Whole grains
Barley, whole or pearled
Bread, whole-grain
Brown rice
Cereal, whole-grain
Crackers, whole-grain
Millet
Oatmeal
Pasta, wheat
Rolls, whole-grain
Wild rice

MEDIUM SATIETY

Fruits
Apricots
Bananas
Cantaloupe
Cherries
Dried fruit (prunes, raisins)
Grapefruit
Grapes, green, purple, red
Honeydew
Kiwifruit
Mangoes

Nectarines
Papayas
Peaches
Plums
Pomegranates
Tangerines
Watermelon

Whole grains
Amaranth
Buckwheat groats (kasha)
Bulgur
Kashi
Popcorn, air-popped without butter
Quinoa
Rye, whole kernel
Wheat, whole kernel

Low Satiety

Bread, white
Cake
Candy, all kinds
Candy bars
Cookies
Crackers, prepared with white flour
Croissants
Doughnuts
French fries
Ice cream
Low-fat baked goods
Muffins
Potato chips
Pretzels

3 | Get Started on the Fill Up to Slim Down Plan

There's nothing magical about weight loss: Burn more calories than you take in and the pounds will drop off. That said, there *are* practical, commonsense strategies that can make your weight-loss journey easier and more pleasant. Below you'll find dozens of tips that can give you the edge while you're following the Fill Up to Slim Down way of eating. Use them in good health!

Cooking for Fullness

Low-fat cooking can be easy and tasty, once you learn a few simple guidelines. Follow these tips for surefire success:

- Use healthy, low-fat cooking methods, such as broiling, steaming, roasting, grilling, poaching, and stir-frying. Remember, though—these methods are low-fat only if you don't add fat while cooking.
- Cook only with lean cuts of beef, pork, lamb, and poultry. Loin and round cuts have less fat. Trim all visible fat and remove the skin before cooking.
- Flavor food with herbs, spices, marinades, salsa, flavored vinegars, and fat-free salad dressing, rather than butter, margarine, or oil. The table on pages 39–40 can help you find the perfect spice, regardless of what you're preparing.
- Chill soups and stews and skim off the fat before you eat them.
- Drain and rinse cooked ground beef under hot water before you add it to spaghetti sauce, tacos, or similar recipes.
- Use nonstick skillets to reduce the amount of liquid or fat needed to keep food from sticking in the pan.
- To soak up extra fat, use paper liners in muffin pans and parchment on baking sheets.
- Spray your pasta pot with cooking spray before you boil pasta—it will keep the noodles from sticking.
- Applesauce can stand in for half to one-third of the fat called for in recipes.
- Plain low-fat or fat-free yogurt is an excellent substitute for sour cream. You can also use half fat-free sour cream and half light sour cream for fuller flavor and fewer fat calories. Try it on your next baked potato.
- Chew gum while you cook, so you don't end up "tasting" hundreds of extra calories.
- Or munch on cut-up veggies while you cook. It's a great way to keep yourself from tasting, and it helps you get in your veggies for the day.

PRACTICE "SAFE PORTIONS"

Knowing the size of a serving is crucial to portion control, and therefore to weight loss. To get an idea of what a serving looks like, imagine these equivalents:

3 ounces chicken or fish	Deck of cards
1 cup vegetables	Size of your fist
Medium apple	Size of a baseball
½ cup pasta, cooked	Ice cream scoop or tennis ball
1½ ounces cheese	Pair of dice or pair of dominoes
1 tablespoon butter/margarine	thumbtip
¼ cup dry cereal	Large egg
1 cup salad greens	Size of a fist
1 baked potato	Size of a fist
1½ ounces natural cheese	Size of 3 dominoes
1 ounce processed cheese	Size of 4 dice
2 tablespoons peanut butter	Size of a golf ball
3 ounces grilled/baked fish	Size of a checkbook
2 tablespoons salad dressing	Size of a Ping-Pong ball
1 ounce of nuts	2 shot glasses
1 ounce chips or pretzels	Cupped handful
A large bagel	Size of a hockey puck
Cup of lettuce	Four leaves
1 pancake	Size of a compact disc
Steamed rice	Cupcake wrapper
¼ cup sour cream	Golf ball

Your Shopping Guide

If you don't bring unhealthy, high-fat foods in the house, you probably won't eat them. Here's how to make sure you come home from the supermarket with foods that support your weight-loss goals.

- Never shop when you're hungry. You'd be surprised at the sugary, fatty foods that find their way into your cart!
- If fresh veggies tend to rot in your crisper, buy frozen vegetables instead. They're still full of fiber and nutrients, and you can just toss them into stir-fries or put them on top of whole-grain pasta.
- Switch to 1-percent or fat-free milk and lower-fat cheeses, particularly those made from part-skim milk such as low-fat or fat-free mozzarella, ricotta, or cream cheese.
- Look for low-fat cuts of meat. "Select" cuts are lower in fat than "prime" and "choice."
- Ground turkey breast is much lower in fat than regular ground turkey.
- Tuna packed in water has fewer fat calories than tuna packed in oil.
- Choose low-fat or non-fat versions of your favorite salad dressings, mayonnaise, yogurt, and sour cream. If you really dislike the flavor of the fat-free versions, mix the fat-free kinds with the light versions.
- Choose low-fat or "lite" tub margarine instead of butter or stick margarine. However, even these spreads are a concentrated source of fat, so use them in moderation. Look for margarines that do not list trans fat as an ingredient on the label.
- Use fat-free jams and preserves, or Butter Buds or fat-free spray butter, instead of butter, margarine, or cream cheese.

Don't Go Supplement Crazy

Healthy people who eat a healthy diet of at least 1,200 to 1,400 calories a day generally obtain the vitamins and minerals their bodies need, including vitamin C. But for extra insurance, consider taking a daily multivitamin/mineral supplement.

The multi you choose should have 100 percent of the Daily Value (DV) of most essential vitamins and minerals and get part or all of its vitamin A as beta-carotene, which the body uses to make vitamin A. Too much vitamin A may cause bone fractures in postmenopausal women and is linked to birth defects. Also, if you're a woman, consider taking the three supplements below.

Calcium. It's important to meet the recommended amount of this mineral—1,000 milligrams if you're premenopausal, 1,500 milligrams a day if postmenopausal—because inadequate calcium intake is linked to osteoporosis. If you don't get enough calcium from dairy products and leafy green vegetables, consider taking a supplement. Avoid those made from bone meal, oyster shell, or dolomite, which may be contaminated with heavy metals. Instead, choose supplements with calcium citrate or calcium carbonate. To increase the amount of calcium you absorb, take calcium in divided doses throughout the day.

Folic acid. If you're pregnant or planning to be, be sure to get at least 400 micrograms of folic acid—also called folate—per day to help prevent birth defects. While you may get enough folate through food, ask your doctor about taking a supplement as extra nutritional insurance.

Iron. Iron is an important component of hemoglobin, the compound in blood that carries oxygen to organs and muscles. Iron deficiency can result in anemia, which causes weakness, shortness of breath, lack of energy, and mental fogginess.

The RDA of iron for women ages thirty-one to fifty is 18 milligrams a day; ages fifty-one and over, 8 milligrams a day; pregnant women, 27 milligrams a day. While one of the best sources of iron is lean meat, fish, poultry, whole grains, dried beans, peas, lentils, and green leafy vegetables are also good sources. To increase the body's absorption of iron, serve iron-rich foods with foods that are high in vitamin C.

If you're premenopausal and you eat little or no meat or cereal, ask your doctor if you might benefit from taking an iron supplement or a multi that contains iron. If you're postmenopausal, skip the supplement—research has linked high iron levels at this stage of life with an increased risk of heart disease.

Snacking

Eating every three to four hours keeps blood sugar levels steady and curbs that ravenous sensation. That's where snacks come in. Healthy snacks provide essential nutrients and keep blood insulin levels stable. To indulge in "smart snacking," follow the tips below.

- Most people snack at around the same time each day. Do you? If so, make this snack a part of your daily food plan, and plan ahead for what to eat.
- Snack to feel full, not to feel stuffed. Your next meal is just an hour or two away.
- Make some of your favorite snacks part of your daily meal plan. Balance high-fat or high-calorie snacks with low-calorie and low-fat choices at other meals, or with other snacks. Don't forbid your favorites—you'll only crave them more.
- Snack consciously. Focus on what you're eating, not on your magazine or TV show.
- Try eating fruit at room temperature instead of cold from the refrigerator. Most fruits taste sweeter and closer to "fresh off the tree" when they are allowed to warm up a bit, as they would be beneath a summer sun.
- Many people confuse hunger and thirst. Before you reach for food, reach for a cold glass of water, sugar-free lemonade, or iced herbal tea. Or make flavored water by mixing three-fourths cup plain or sparkling water with one-fourth cup fruit juice.
- Place binge-trigger foods in hard-to-reach places and keep them inside opaque containers. What the eye doesn't see, it often doesn't desire.

Top Snack Foods

UNDER 100 CALORIES	UNDER 200 CALORIES
1 cup fat-free yogurt or pudding	1 low-fat flour tortilla + 2 tablespoons nonfat refried beans + 1 to 2 tablespoons chunky-style salsa
1 cup dry, unsweetened cereal	1 cup low-fat vegetable soup + 5 saltine crackers
1 cup unsweetened applesauce sprinkled with cinnamon	1 cup Corn Chex + ½ cup skim milk + ¼ cup blueberries
1 slice fat-free bread with 1 teaspoon fruit preserves	2 ounces low-fat deli turkey on 5 mini rice cakes
1 sourdough English muffin with 1 teaspoon fruit preserves	2 cups air-popped popcorn + ¼ cup raisins
10 jelly beans (regular) or 25 Jelly Belly candies	3-inch cinnamon raisin bagel with 1 tablespoon light or nonfat cream cheese
4 ounces frozen fruit sorbet	4 mini rice cakes with 4 teaspoons peanut butter
2 fat-free Fig Newtons	1 cup nonfat cottage cheese + 4 whole-wheat crackers
1 hard pretzel	½ cup nonfat chocolate sorbet with ½ cup sliced banana and 2 teaspoons chocolate syrup
1 fat-free fudge pop	¾ cup low-fat cottage cheese with ½ cup pineapple chunks
1 apple or orange	½ pita and ¼ cup hummus
1 cup strawberries	1 cup cooked brown rice flavored with 3 tablespoons salsa
2 kiwifruit	1 slice whole-wheat toast spread with 1 tablespoon peanut butter and 2 teaspoons honey

(continued)

Under 100 Cal	Under 200 Cal
1 frozen fruit-juice bar	½ cup chocolate low-fat frozen yogurt plus ½ cup fresh or frozen berries
2 flavored rice cakes	Turkey sandwich (2 slices whole-wheat bread, 4 slices deli thin turkey breast, 1 slice tomato, 2 teaspoons mustard)
3 cups air-popped popcorn	
1 celery stalk stuffed with 1 tablespoon fat-free cream cheese	

Spice Up Your Life

If you have high blood pressure, your doctor will recommend that you reduce your intake of sodium. The most common source of dietary sodium is table salt. One teaspoon contains 2,300 milligrams, and Americans typically consume 6,000 to 12,000 milligrams each day.

Limiting salt does not doom you to a life of tasteless food. Use the table below to experiment with herbs, spices, and other seasonings to enhance the natural flavors of foods. Consider planting a windowsill herb garden, so you can have fresh herbs all year long.

Spice	Use
Allspice	baked goods, puddings, and fruit, takes the place of cinnamon, cloves, and nutmeg
Basil leaves	fish, salads, all tomato-based dishes, soups, salad dressings, dips
Bay leaves	soups, stews, other long-cooking dishes—but always remove them before serving

(continued)

Spice	Use
Celery seed	breads, vegetables, and meat dishes
Chili powder	chili and meat sauces
Chives	potatoes, vegetables, salads
Cinnamon	cooked fruits, winter squash, baked goods
Cloves	baked goods, puddings, soups, cooked fruits, teas or cider, winter squash
Cumin seed	curry dishes, soups, chili, all Mexican-style recipes
Curry powder	vegetable dishes
Dill	baked goods, cheese dishes
Fennel	Use roasted bulb in pasta sauces and rice
Ginger	cooked fruits, chicken, stir-fry, sweet potatoes, pumpkin, carrots, baked goods such as gingerbread or pumpkin pie
Marjoram	Fish, meat, poultry, stuffing, soups, and stews
Nutmeg	Baked goods, pumpkin, sweet potatoes, carrots, soups
Oregano	pizzas, Italian-style dishes (especially pastas), vegetables, dips, fish, salads, soups
Paprika	chilis, veggie stews
Parsley	soup, salad, vegetables, potatoes, garnishes for any dish
Rosemary	fish, meat, poultry, stuffing, vegetables, potatoes, stews
Sage	soups, stews, stuffing, salad dressings, fish, pizza sauce
Tarragon	good in most Italian-style dishes, also on vegetables
Thyme	tomato-based dishes, soups, sauces, salad dressings, poultry seasoning, herbed breads

Thinking the Fill Up to Slim Down Way

While you focus on what you're putting into your mouth and on your plate, give some thought to what's in your head, too. Fact is, your thoughts can help your progress—or hinder it. The tips below can help you think about food and eating in healthy, helpful ways.

- Practice HALT—be extra careful around food when you're Hungry, Angry, Lonely, or Tired.
- If you want to eat outside of a meal or snack, ask yourself whether you're really physically hungry or bored, angry, lonely, or blue. If you're not sure, don't eat until you experience physical symptoms of hunger, such as light-headedness, headache, or a rumbly stomach.
- Take the TV out of your kitchen so that you're aware of how much you eat.
- Eat at least one or two dinners a week at a table set with your "good dishes" and without the background noise of the television or radio—even if you live alone. Make these meals events—flowers on the table, cloth napkins, the works.
- When you find yourself picking, go brush your teeth. It gets you out of harm's way, and when your mouth is fresh and clean, you're less likely to nibble.
- Don't think of foods as "good" or "bad." Instead, think of them as "more healthy" and "less healthy." Remember, a truly healthy diet is all about balance, portion control, and variety.
- Think positive. Get your attitude in shape and your body will follow.
- Slipping up doesn't mean you have to give up. If you eat more than you would have liked one day, recommit to the Fill Up to Slim Down way of eating the next.

4 Eating Out the Fill Up to Slim Down Way

Many of us spend a good portion of our days on the road, eating on the run. You're at the mercy of restaurants, airlines, and fast-food joints—right?

The truth is, eating away from home can be as healthful as it is tasty and fun—if you make wise choices. The principles of smart eating that guide your food choices at home still apply to the meals you eat away from home. These principles include ordering low-fat versions of your favorite items, making substitutions, and making specific requests to your servers or the cook.

In fact, eating healthy while dining out has become a whole lot easier. Most restaurants—even the fast-food joints!—have heeded the public's interest in healthier cuisine and now offer a wide variety of heart-healthy, waistline-conscious fare. In fact, many offer meals that are lower in fat, cholesterol, sodium, and calories, often marked as such on the menu.

The bottom line? No matter where you dine—from the greasiest of greasy spoons to the fanciest four-star restaurant—you're bound to find items on the menu that meet guidelines for the Fill Up to Slim Down way of eating, such as fresh fruits and veggies, lean proteins, and healthy complex carbohydrates. You may have to look for these items, but they're there. This chapter can help guide you through virtually any menu so you can make healthier choices.

OUTWIT YOUR APPETITE

Here are some good general guidelines for ordering a meal.

- Review the menu carefully to see what's available. These days, you can often check out a menu online; if not, call ahead. If you don't see what you need or want, ask if you can have something similar but prepared more simply.
- Give specific cooking instructions and ask for food to be prepared without salt, butter, cream, or excess oil. This doesn't mean you'll be eating food that contains none of these. It's possible, even likely, that restaurant foods will contain "hidden" fats, but don't let that discourage you. The goal isn't perfection, just to minimize unwanted fats in favor of healthier preparations.
- If you feel embarrassed to be making special requests, change the emphasis in your mind to one of your health concerns. Someone with allergies wouldn't hesitate to mention that to the server; decide that you're in a similar situation. As one of my patients once commented, "I'm allergic to butter—I break out in fat!"
- Order salad dressings and sauces on the side. That way, you control exactly how much you consume. You may decide to eat every last ounce of the sauce or dressing you're served, but it will be *your* choice.
- Buy a small cooler and pack healthy snacks you can nibble on at your desk at work and in your car, such as low-fat cheese sticks,

(continued)

cut-up veggies and dip, grapes and other "finger fruit," or a handful of heart-healthy nuts (no more than a handful, though). If you never get too hungry, you won't be susceptible to making unhealthy fast-food choices.

Breakfast: Wake Up to Healthy Options

Most fast-food breakfast items are high in fat and calories and low in satisfaction—that is, they're mostly fat, sodium, and junk carbohydrates like white flour and sugar, with little or no fiber or good-for-you whole grains. If you must go through the drive-through, avoid the breakfast sandwiches and muffins and opt for eggs. If you can, order breakfast at a diner or coffee shop, which usually offers more and better options.

Fruit. Select any fresh fruit (berries, bananas, melon) or choose canned fruits packed in fruit juice or water instead of syrup. To really fill your stomach, opt for whole fruit, if it's offered, instead of juice.

Cereal. Hot or cold cereals such as oatmeal, Cream of Wheat, Raisin Bran, and shredded wheat are good choices. Use reduced-fat or non-fat milk and ask your server for a side of sliced fruit or applesauce—both sweeten hot cereal just fine. Request that hot cereals not be prepared with whole milk or butter.

Eggs and other proteins. If you opt for eggs, limit egg yolks to four per week. Or look for items made with egg substitute or egg whites—the newer substitutes are just as tasty as the real thing. Stuff an omelette with veggies instead of cheese. For a side, choose Canadian bacon, lean turkey, or chicken sausage instead of regular bacon or sausage.

Bagels, muffins, and other breakfast breads. As a rule, the common bagel isn't a great choice—they're usually very large and made with unhealthy white flour—and many muffins are high in fat, calories, and sugar. A plain bran or corn muffin is your best bet.

Better options: half a whole-grain bagel, or whole-grain wheat or rye toast. Spread them with a very small amount of fruit spread or low-fat cream cheese, if it's offered, instead of butter or full-fat cream cheese. Skip French toast, doughnuts, and other pastries, including croissants— they contain outrageous amounts of fat and/or sugar.

DE-FAT FAST FOOD

While some fast-food chains offer lighter items, such as salads and grilled chicken, the majority of menu items contain huge amounts of fat and calories. These guidelines can help de-fat and fiber-up a fast-food meal.

- Frequent fast-food chains that offer grilled chicken salads or baked potatoes. If you order a spud, skip the high-fat, high-calorie toppings, or ask for them on the side.
- Order smaller portions. For example, opt for one small hamburger instead of a double, or a small fries instead of a large.
- Hold the sauces!
- Limit high-fat, high-calorie burger toppings and condiments, such as bacon, cheese, mayonnaise, sauces, and dressings.
- Choose broiled or grilled chicken sandwiches over the fried versions, and hold the sauces.
- Limit or avoid french fries, ham, sausage, bacon, and cheese.
- Avoid milk shakes and dessert items such as pies and sundaes.

Lunch and Dinner: Sit Down to These Hearty, Healthy Choices

Lunch presents a variety of challenges. If you're required to entertain at lunch, pick restaurants where you can get what you want and need, and become a regular. A staff that knows your wishes reduces the stress that dining out can produce.

If you're a regular at the company cafeteria, decide in advance what you want to eat so that you're not distracted or tempted by specials that may be high in fat, calories, and sodium. Your best bet may be the salad bar or made-to-order sandwiches prepared with lean meats and reduced-fat cheeses. If you'd like to see more healthy options, ask: you're surely not the only one requesting healthier fare.

Dining out in the evening need not derail healthy eating. Most restaurants will honor reasonable requests for substitutions or preparation methods; their business depends on satisfied customers. Don't be afraid to ask your server about items on the menu, or to discuss substitutions. Also, keep in mind that not every dinner out is a celebration or occasion. Most of the time, it's just dinner—don't take it as carte blanche to overindulge.

Here's help in wading through your lunch and dinner options.

Appetizers. A well-chosen appetizer can help you stick to your plan. It will satisfy your initial hunger, so you won't feel ravenous when the entrée is served, and you'll find it easier to eat less of the main course. A tossed salad made of leafy greens and other raw vegetables is an excellent choice, as are fresh fruit salads. Ask for fat-free or low-fat salad dressing served on the side, or use salsa, vinegar, or lemon juice. Fruit juice, melon, raw vegetables, or shrimp cocktail are also excellent choices.

Bread. By all means, enjoy *one* piece of bread or a roll before your meal if you wish. But after you take a piece, ask your server to remove the bread basket, or send it to the other end of the table. Or eat it "naked"; really good bread doesn't need anything on top.

Soup. Choose clear soups such as bouillon or consommé or broth-based vegetable soups. Gazpacho is a good choice in the warmer months. Avoid cream soups.

Sandwiches and wraps. Choose turkey or lean ham, which contain only 1 to 2 grams of fat per ounce, or a grilled burger made with lean ground beef or turkey. Skip the bologna or salami, which contain up to 8 grams of fat per ounces, as well as mayo-laden tuna or shrimp salads. To slash saturated fat, order sandwiches without cheese, bacon, oil, or mayonnaise. (Or ask for mayo on the side and use it sparingly.) Substitute healthier condiments. Use mustard rather than mayonnaise, or pepper or lemon juice instead of salt. Avoid bologna, salami, pastrami, or corned beef, as well as open-faced sandwiches served with gravy.

Salads. If you order a Caesar salad, get the dressing and the Parmesan cheese on the side, so you can control the amount you're eating. Instead, choose a spinach, seafood, grilled chicken, or fresh fruit salad, low-fat or reduced-fat dressing on the side. Order dressing on the side and dab your fork in the sauce and then spear your salad.

At salad bars, choose raw vegetables, leafy greens, beans, and fresh fruit. Avoid high-fat items such as deli meats, egg yolk, bacon, and most cheeses, as well as cole slaw, potato salad, and macaroni salad. Nuts, croutons, and other crunchy toppings, such as chow mein noodles or bacon bits, should be labeled "handle with care." Have a tablespoonful, no more. Choose dressings with care; one ladleful may contain several hundred calories and lots of unhealthy fat.

Entrées. Restaurant dining can be a good time to choose foods you don't always make at home, especially fish. Avoid breaded or fried meats, opting instead for 3-ounce portions of lean beef, pork, or poultry, roasted, broiled, or grilled. (A 3-ounce serving of meat should fit in the palm of your hand or be the size of a deck of playing cards.) Order meat and fish broiled without added butter and/or salt. Most chefs are used to such requests and will usually moisten the food with a squeeze of lemon or lime juice or a splash of wine. When your entrée arrives, cut away visible fat.

Side dishes. Steamed or grilled vegetables without butter and little oil are always good choices as are brown rice and potatoes (baked, broiled, or roasted) served without butter or sour cream. A baked sweet potato is a real treat if they're offered, as are roasted vegetables. Avoid french fries, potato chips, onion rings, or mayonnaise-based salads.

Beverages. Besides water, fruit and veggie juices, and diet sodas, you may enjoy sparkling water, unsweetened iced tea, coffee, and black or green tea, lightened with fat-free milk or fat-free half-and-half and sweetened with artificial sweeteners instead of heaping teaspoonfuls of sugar.

If you're drinking alcoholic beverages, drink them in moderation—alcohol can stimulate appetite and reduce inhibitions about overeating. Avoid mixed drinks made with soft drinks, coconut milk, or presweetened mixes, such as piña coladas or frozen daiquiris. Ask that your margarita be made without salt, or limit yourself to one and watch your sodium the rest of the day.

Dessert. Choose fresh fruit, nonfat or low-fat frozen yogurt, sorbet, sherbet, sugar-free gelatin, or a low-fat cake such as angel food. What about chocolate? Recent studies have suggested that dark chocolate has heart-protective qualities, but more research is needed to ascertain just how good for you it may be. In the meantime, chocolate should be viewed as a special occasion food—when you splurge, choose the best dark chocolate you can afford.

HIGH-FLYING FOODS

When you're trapped 30,000 feet up for five or six hours and you're ravenous, it's easy to say, "Well, I'll eat whatever I'm served." But you don't have to, if you plan ahead.

All major airlines provide meals that conform to specific dietary needs—at no extra cost. A recent check of the United Airlines Web site, for example, found that it serves diabetic, high-fiber, low-calorie, low fat/low-cholesterol, low-protein, and low-sodium options, usually with twenty-four to forty-eight hours' notice (check with your airline to be sure). You can also opt for a fruit plate or several different kinds of vegetarian meals (though these may not be as low in fat as you might prefer).

The good news is that these meals are better now than they used to be. Gone are the days of the dry chicken breast and limp iceberg lettuce. Now you're more likely to dine on a whole grain roll with reduced-fat margarine, an appetizer of shrimp on a bed of lettuce with spicy cocktail sauce, and roast chicken and vegetables, rice, or pasta. (Give away the desserts, though, unless it's a low-fat or low-calorie version of a high-fat favorite.)

Making Ethnic Healthy Again

Excess calories, fat, and sodium can find their way into ethnic cuisine, too, especially when it's prepared American-style. Here's how to make the smartest choices, whatever your favorite ethnic cuisine.

Chinese. Fortunately, many Chinese dishes contain high-fiber, low-fat ingredients such as vegetables and grains. Look for stir-fried (request little or no oil) or steamed dishes that contain lean beef, chicken, seafood, vegetables, or tofu (also known as bean curd) dishes. Request brown rice, if it's available. Skip the sweet-and-sour sauce and typical fried items such as egg rolls, wontons, fried rice, and fried noodles. To limit sodium, ask that your food be prepared without added salt, monosodium glutamate (MSG), or soy sauce. If you love garlic sauce, have it, but order it on the side and simply dip steamed chicken and vegetables in the sauce.

Indian. The spices used in Indian dishes add flavor without fat, and the cuisine includes lots of legumes and lentils. The best choices include chicken or fish prepared tandoori-style, legume-based dishes (called dals), rice-based dishes (biryanis), and baked bread (naan). Avoid fried breads, fried entrées, and dishes prepared with coconut cream.

Italian. Pasta is at the center of many Italian dishes, and although it's made with white flour, at least it's low in fat. Red or white clam sauces and fresh tomato-based sauces like marinara are good choices, as are grilled, broiled, or roasted fish or chicken. Avoid dairy-based sauces such as Alfredo sauce and baked dishes that are topped with cheese (like baked ziti). Also avoid items with pancetta or prosciutto (Italian bacon and ham), which are high in sodium. Ask the chef to use wine instead of butter to sauté your entrée, and start your meal with a large salad dressed with low-fat or fat-free dressing, served on the side.

Mexican. Eating Mexican usually presents a challenge, as many typical Mexican foods contain saturated fat, but you can find a healthy dish among the fat bombs. First, skip the fried chips that are usually served before the meal. Choose items that are baked rather than fried. Your best choices include soft tacos and burritos filled with white-meat chicken, beans (made without lard), and/or rice, with little or no cheese. (Request corn tortillas in place of lard-based flour tortillas.) Or opt for a fajita, which usually contains grilled onions and peppers. Avoid fried foods (crispy tacos, nachos, tostada shells, flautas, chimichangas), refried beans and tortillas made with lard, quesadillas, and the extras—cheese, guacamole, and sour cream (if you must, choose one rather than all three). Choose black beans and plain rice instead. Use salsa and hot sauce for added flavor.

Eating American

Eating American often means eating big—big slabs of meat, oversized platters groaning with fat-soaked appetizers, huge pizzas stuffed with meat and cheese. And yet, you can find healthy offerings, even at the large chain restaurants. To give your heart—and your waistline—a break, follow these simple guidelines.

Steak houses. If you must have red meat, order filet mignon, flank steak, or London broil—all are lean cuts of beef. Enjoy 3 ounces, or have 6 ounces and have non-meat entrées the rest of the day. (You might consider sharing a portion of 10 ounces or more with a dining companion.) However, your best bet is to order broiled or baked fish, skinless chicken, game hen, or turkey, prepared without extra fats like butter or gravy. A baked potato, brown/wild rice, and/or a salad and steamed vegetables, prepared without added fat, are excellent side dishes.

Chicken joints. Choose rotisserie or grilled chicken over fried. Remove the skin to significantly reduce fat and calories, and select white meat over dark. Choose lower-fat side dishes such as barbecue beans, a baked sweet potato, oven-roasted potatoes, corn, squash, green beans, or a green salad. Avoid gravies, vegetables smothered in cheese or cream sauces, and potato or macaroni salads.

Pizza parlors. The inventor of the cheese-stuffed crust may have scored a marketing success, but muster all your willpower and avoid it—it's the unhealthiest pizza selection you can make. To save your arteries, choose thin crust over thick, choose vegetable toppings over meats like pepperoni, ham, and sausage, and order a side salad instead of chowing down on those one or two extra slices.

Pare down those portions!

Most restaurants serve oversized portions of just about everything—appetizers, pasta, meat, dessert. This means oversized portions of calories, fat, cholesterol, and sodium. Here's how to watch "portion creep."

- Ask if you can have a lunch portion, even at dinner. If the restaurant won't allow this, ask that they place half the food in a to-go container and the other half on your plate.
- Split a meal with a dining partner.
- Eat only until your hunger is satisfied. If you're tempted to clean your plate, ask your server to remove the dishes.
- Avoid buffets, if possible. If you can't, examine the entire buffet *first,* then decide what you want and take only that.

5 | Your Weight-Loss Tool Kit

As you embark upon your weight-loss journey, the tools in this chapter can help you reach your destination: a healthy weight. Some will be familiar, while others may be new to you. But they all have one thing in common: Used consistently, they can be a core part of your success. While you don't have to use any of them, we encourage you to be adventurous and try a tool you haven't before. It may be the one that helps you keep off the weight for good!

Tool #1: A Weight-Loss Journal

Keeping a journal while you're on the Fill Up to Slim Down program is a great way to track your progress. Depending on what you wish to include in your journal (see below), you can use a fancy leather diary, a small, purse-sized spiral notebook, a composition book or three-ring binder, or even an online diet and fitness journal, such as www.fitday.com.

What should your journal include? These ideas will help get you started.

- A running account of what you eat throughout the day. Writing down what, when, and why you eat can help you understand the factors that influence your eating patterns. Don't worry about making it pretty, just scribble the information as you go.
- How many grams of healthy fiber and satisfying complex carbohydrates you consume (aim for between 20 and 35 grams of fiber per day). You may want to purchase a calorie counter that includes fiber grams.
- Your daily water intake. (Because you'll be consuming significantly more fiber, aim for between eight and ten glasses a day.)
- Your daily exercise—what you did, and for how long. You may even want to include what you thought about during or after your workout. Were you aware of new strength, a quicker recovery to your resting heartbeat, a glow on your cheeks? By all means, write it down!
- Quotes, pictures, or articles that inspire you.
- Pictures of yourself that allow you to see the progress you have made.

Many people's weight-loss journals include their thoughts and feelings about their weight-loss program. Write for a page or a dozen, as the spirit moves you. And write about anything you wish. Write about your health concerns and fears, your past failures and your past successes. Record how proud you are on days that you excel, as well as how you conquered any challenges that day. Reflect on how you are feeling as you contemplate this new beginning.

To pull up a sample journal page, log onto Jyl's Web site, www. americashealthiestmom.com.

TAKE A LOOK BACK: THE WEEKLY ROUNDUP

Including a weekly roundup in your journal is a good way to review what occurred during the past seven days. By reflecting on what's working for you, and troubleshooting what isn't, you can determine how the next week will go. Here are some issues you might explore on a weekly basis.

- What were some of your triumphs this week? Did you resist a craving to stop for an ice cream cone? Say no to a colleague's homemade chocolate chip cookies? This is your time to brag—writing down your successes may actually help you replicate them.
- What were some of your challenges? Did you feel down one night and give in to your yearning for potato chips? Binge after a confrontation with your boss? Brainstorm ideas on how you might address these issues next time they occur.
- What do you want to see next week? Is there a specific goal you want to aim for—a new food to try, more weight on a barbell, or getting more sleep?
- What was the best meal or recipe you had this week? Why did you enjoy it?

SET "SMART" GOALS

Well-written goals are among your most helpful tools. By admitting what you want, you're already on your way to making it happen. Design your written goals (remember to be SMART when setting goals):

Specific. State exactly what you want to achieve, how you plan to do it, and when you want to achieve it. At first, set goals that you can achieve in a week or two—it's easy to give up on goals that seem too far away. If you have a big goal, break it down into a series of smaller weekly or daily goals. After you achieve one of the smaller goals, move on to the next.

Measurable. A goal that doesn't have some way of measuring whether you've achieved it is useless. "I want to lose weight" can't be measured. But, "I want to lose twenty-five pounds in five months" can.

Attainable. Is your goal reasonable? Be honest! If you've just started jogging, it's unreasonable to assume that you'll finish a marathon that's only three months away. However, you may be able to complete a 5K.

Realistic. Your goals need to be within your capabilities. Set goals that require you to stretch yourself, but that are not completely out of your reach.

Time Oriented. Set a time frame that you want to achieve your goals by. Set short-, medium-, and long-term goals.

Below are examples of SMART goals.

- **Short-term SMART Goal:** In two weeks, I will walk one mile in twenty minutes or less.
- **Mid-term SMART Goal:** I will complete twenty half-hour sessions of aerobic exercise three times a week for three months.
- **Long-term SMART Goal:** In six months, I will enter and run my first community walk or run.

Tool #2: A Pedometer

A pedometer is a device the size of a pager that records the number of steps you take. Research has found that people who use pedometers tend to stay with their exercise program longer. What's more, in a study reported in the *Journal of the American Medical Association,* participants in a healthy lifestyle program who wore pedometers increased their activity levels by about thirty minutes, five days per week, and lost weight—doing nothing but inserting short "activity bursts" into their days!

The average person accumulates 3,000 to 5,000 steps per day. The goal is to increase your number of steps per day to about 10,000. Just a few changes in your routine will help you get those steps in. Here are some ideas, just to get you started.

- Park your car farther away from the door at the shopping center or at your office.
- Use the stairs instead of the elevator.
- On long drives take frequent rest stops to walk for fifteen minutes or so.
- Instead of killing time while waiting for an appointment, take a walk.

Some pedometers simply measure steps, while other, fancier models track the distance you walk and the calories you burn. Basic step counters cost about $20, while more sophisticated models can be $40 or more. Both are available at sporting goods stores.

Tool #3: A Tape Measure

Hate stepping on the scale? Then here's some good news: It's now known that the true measure of health and fitness is body composition—the ratio of body fat to lean muscle tissue. You could go to a gym and get your body fat measured, but it's simpler—and cheaper—to use a plain old cloth tape measure. Here's where to measure:

- chest around the widest part. (For women, you may want to take measurements across the middle of the breast as well as below the breast. As body fat is reduced, you may see a reduction in both of these measurements as well as bra cup size.)
- waist around your natural waistline. If you don't think you have one, then simply pick a point that crosses the navel.
- hips across the fleshiest part of your rear end.
- upper thigh

- calf
- upper arm
- neck (men)

Measure once a month, and keep a record of your measurements in your weight-loss journal. Often you'll see changes in your body that aren't reflected on the scale. Those reductions can be inspiring and encouraging, so give this tool a try.

DON'T BE SCARED OF YOUR SCALE

Anyone who's struggled with weight probably shares the same uncomfortable memories of standing on a doctor's scale, waiting without breathing for those clunky weights to be shifted and deliver the bad news.

Scales have earned a bad rap, getting blamed for the feelings of insecurity and inferiority their numbers inspire. It's time to take the power back. That means using the scale simply as a tool to measure your body, not yourself. Fill Up to Slim Down eating will help you get healthy, and when you add regular exercise to your daily "diet," your scale will reflect the effects of those lifestyle changes.

But it may not deliver them on a perfectly reliable schedule. That doesn't mean you should toss your scale into the nearest landfill or donate it to Goodwill. It just means that you need to use it differently and less often.

There's no value in weighing yourself more than once a week. Daily weight fluctuations are normal and common, so don't let them dissuade you from sticking to your plans for eating and exercise. Also, while the scale shows weight loss of water and fat, it may also show weight gain as you build muscle.

Should you weigh yourself *less often* than once a week? Sure, why not? Perhaps you've developed such an antipathy for the scale that you choose to weigh in every two weeks instead, or even once a month. If you're a woman, you may find you're at your lightest right after your period. If you've passed

(continued)

into menopause, you may still find that you experience cycles during the month that influence your weight.

Use the scale as part of your Weekly Roundup or make it a once-a-month update in your journal. And remember that it's only *one* measurement of your progress toward optimum health.

Tool #4: The Nutrition Facts Label

Listed on the side panel of packaged foods, the Nutrition Facts label is a great way to "comparison-shop" for nutrients—for example, to see which brand of bread or breakfast cereal is higher in fiber. Here's a "cheat sheet."

Serving Size. This refers to the standard size based on amounts people actually eat. Pay attention to the serving size, including how many servings the box, bag, or package actually contains. It may save you from eating many more servings than you want!

- Look at the number of calories per serving, including how many calories are from fat.

Percent Daily Value. Based on dietary recommendations for healthy people, the percent daily value—which indicates how food fits within a 2,000-calorie diet—helps you to understand if the food is a good or not-so-great source of important nutrients. To consume more fiber, vitamins, and minerals, and less saturated fat, cholesterol, and sodium, all you have to do is look at the percentage DV.

- As a rule of thumb, foods with 5 percent of the DV or less contribute a small amount of that nutrient to your diet, while those with 20 percent or more contribute a large amount.

Middle Section. The nutrients listed in the middle section are the ones most important to good health. This helps you calculate your daily limits for fat, fiber, sodium, and other nutrients.

- Limit these nutrients: total fat, including saturated and trans fat, cholesterol, and sodium.

Vitamins and Minerals. The percent daily value is the same as the U.S. recommended daily allowance for vitamins and minerals. Only these vitamins and minerals are required on labels, although the manufacturer has the option to include others.

- Get plenty of fiber, vitamins, calcium, and iron.

Tool #5: A Good Pair of Walking Shoes

If you walk for your cardiovascular exercise, as millions of Americans do, do your feet—and legs—a favor and get a good, sturdy pair of walking shoes. What you wear on your feet can make the difference between an enjoyable walking experience and one marred by sore shins, calluses, or blisters. So before you put foot to path or pavement, check out these tips.

- If you already walk, wear or bring your current walking shoes so the clerk can see how they have worn.
- Go shoe shopping at the end of the day, when your feet are slightly swollen. Also, wear the socks you'll be wearing when you walk.
- Try on both shoes. Your feet may not be the same size (really!).
- When you try them on, you should have about a half-inch of space between your toes and the end of the shoe. You should be able to wiggle your toes freely, but your heel should not slip.
- Give the shoe a good twist. It should be flexible rather than rigid.
- Once you buy your shoes, wear them in the house for a day or two. Don't walk outside in them until you're sure they feel perfect. If they don't, you'll want to exchange them before you wear them outside.

- Replace walking shoes every 500 miles or so. To extend the life of your shoes, wear them only for your walks.

Tool #6: Your Fill Up to Slim Down Supporters—Offline and On

Ultimately, what you do and how you do is up to you. That's the bottom line. But you have the option of asking for help from the people who support you in your efforts to lose weight and get healthy.

Our advice: Don't try to do it alone. Tell your family and friends about your plans and let them know how they can be most helpful to you. Your kids can help with meal preparation or ride their bikes alongside you when you racewalk. An exercise buddy who agrees to share after-dinner walks or exercise classes can help both of you stick to your schedule. Making a deal with a friend to meet for lunch might just make you less apt to cancel if life gets hectic.

You might also join an online weight-loss support group to get advice, share problems, strategize solutions, and just commiserate! One of the largest online diet programs, eDiets.com, has over 200,000 active members. For about $5 a week, members have access around-the-clock to nutritionists and peer-support chat rooms (in addition to shopping lists, cooking tips, and meal ideas). You can use a site like this to keep your daily log of food and weight loss, if you like. (And if you forget, a message will pop up on your computer the next time you sign on.) This may not work for everyone, but if you've got a complicated schedule, unusual work hours, or live far from friends who might encourage you in person, you might find what you need on the Web!

You don't get extra credit for succeeding on this program if you do it all by yourself, so why choose to? As the popular motivational definition of TEAM promises: Together Everyone Achieves More!

6 Exercise: A Prescription to Last a Lifetime

Exercise is a crucial part of any weight-loss program, and the Fill Up to Slim Down program is no exception. To shed body fat for good, it's not enough simply to eat fewer calories than you burn—you must also burn more calories! It's that simple.

However, exercise isn't important just for weight loss, or even weight maintenance. It's a lifestyle "prescription" for a longer, healthier, and, yes, happier life.

Regular physical activity helps protect you from heart disease, diabetes, cancer, and other chronic diseases. It will also strengthen your immune system, which can help ward off colds, flu, and infection, reduce your risk of osteoporosis, and help you safeguard your ability to care for yourself as you grow older.

Once you make exercise a vital part of your life, you will begin to see remarkable benefits. Your energy level will increase, you'll likely sleep better than you ever have, and you may experience greater pleasure in every physical activity (including lovemaking). Your skin will glow, too, because physical activity improves circulation. And, of course, those extra pounds will begin to melt away.

In fact, regular exercise can make you look as if you've just returned from a great vacation—but you'll know the true secret to your body's new radiance.

To optimize your weight-loss efforts and your overall health, engage in a variety of physical activities. What's more, burning fat doesn't depend solely on how long you work out. Equally important is how *hard* you work out—the intensity of your effort.

Ready to strengthen your heart and lungs while you melt away body fat and stress? To keep up with your kids on the playground? To have some *fun*? Get ready to

Energize and
X-ert yourself for
Excellent
Rewards from
Challenging,
Invigorating, and
Stimulating
EXERCISE!

Your Exercise "Menu"

A comprehensive fitness routine includes three categories of physical activity. The first is cardiovascular exercise, also known as aerobic exercise or "cardio" for short. When you perform aerobic exercise, your heart has to work harder to get oxygen to your muscles, which strengthens your heart and lungs and burns body fat. Cardio includes walking, jogging, bicycling, dancing—any activity that raises your heart rate for at least twenty minutes.

The second type of activity a slim, trim body needs is strength training, also known as resistance training or weightlifting. Strength training revs up your metabolism, which transforms your muscles into powerful fat burners, and firms your muscles, which gives your body a firm, toned appearance. Unlike cardio, strength training is an anaerobic activity, which means that it primarily strengthens your muscles, rather than your heart.

Flexibility exercises (stretching) is the last item on your exercise menu. But it's certainly not least! Stretching exercises—both before and after exercise—improve your ability to move your joints and use muscles through their full range of motion, which keeps your body lithe and limber.

Here's the exercise equation:

$$\text{AEROBIC ACTIVITY + STRENGTH TRAINING}$$
$$\text{+ STRETCHING = FITNESS!}$$

The key to weight loss and good health is to incorporate all three aspects of fitness in your regular workout routine. You don't have to run marathons, climb mountains, or take hours of high-impact step aerobics classes to see results. Physical activity performed at a moderate level of intensity will do your body good—and your mind and spirit, too!

Remember, the "best" exercise routine is the one that works for *you,* that fits your unique schedule, habits, personality, and temperament. Choose an activity that you actually enjoy (tennis, swimming, and roller skating count as cardio!) that fits your budget, along with a convenient time and place.

Get checked by your physician before you begin any exercise program, especially if you have a medical condition that requires special attention, such as heart disease, diabetes, arthritis/joint problems, osteoporosis, dizziness, epilepsy, or pregnancy. If you develop symptoms such as chest pain, palpitations, shortness of breath, dizziness, changes in severity of leg discomfort, or extreme fatigue during exercise, *stop exercising* and notify your doctor immediately.

TWENTY-FIVE BENEFITS OF EXERCISE

1. Strengthens the heart
2. Strengthens the lungs
3. Strengthens the bones
4. Strengthens the muscles
5. Strengthens the joints
6. Strengthens the back
7. Boosts mood
8. Speeds recovery from childbirth
9. Increases "good" (HDL) cholesterol
10. Improves coordination
11. Benefits memory
12. Improves flexibility
13. Increases mobility
14. Speeds metabolic rate
15. Improves sleep
16. Improves posture
17. Boosts energy
18. Improves sex
19. Increases productivity
20. Boosts self-confidence
21. Helps maintain weight loss
22. Helps reduce elevated blood pressure
23. Helps reduce risk of cardiovascular disease, diabetes, and other chronic diseases
24. Helps reduce stress and/or anxiety
25. Helps reduce depression

Fill Up to Slim Down Exercise Prescription 1: Cardio

Adults should engage in cardiovascular exercise three to five times a week for twenty to sixty minutes at a time, according to the American College of Sports Medicine (ACSM). If you haven't been active recently, you might start out with five or ten minutes a day and work up to more time each week. Or split up your daily activity. For example, try a brisk ten-minute walk after each meal.

Here are some other types of cardio you may want to try.

- Walk or jog on a treadmill
- Peddle on a stationary bicycle or elliptical trainer
- Dance (swing dancing is fun and a real calorie-burner!)
- Take a low-impact aerobics class
- Ice- or roller-skate
- Swim
- Stair climb

STEP LIVELY!

Whatever aerobic activity you choose, try to do it for twenty minutes—thirty, if you can. Research indicates that during the first twenty minutes of aerobic activity, the body burns its stored carbohydrates (glycogen), and doesn't burn fat for energy until the glycogen runs out.

Also, make sure that you work at the highest level of effort, or intensity, that feels comfortable to you. To measure intensity during physical activity, check your target heart rate. One way to do it is to subtract your age from 220. Then multiply your result by either 0.6 or 0.9 percent to get your target heart rate range. (If you're under a doctor's care, ask him or her to help you arrive at your ideal heart rate.)

For example, if you're forty years old, you begin with this equation:

$220 - 40 = 180$ hearbeats per minute. To get your lower-limit exercise rate, multiply 180 by 0.6; to get your upper limit, multiply 180 by 0.9. Therefore, your target heart rate ranges from 108 to 162 beats per minute.

If your hearbeats faster than your high-end target, slow down. If it beats fewer than your low-end target, pick up the pace. You'll give your heart a better workout and burn more calories to boot.

Don't have the patience for mathematics? Take the talk-sing test. If you can't talk and exercise at the same time, you're exercising too fast. If you can talk while you exercise, you're doing fine. If you can sing, step lively!

The fitter you get, the faster your heart rate drops after your workout. To determine your resting heart rate, take your pulse immediately after exercise. (The rate decreases rapidly once exercise is slowed or stopped.) You can take your pulse at your wrist or at your neck.

- Wrist: Lightly place the first two fingers of one hand on the thumb side of your other wrist. You will feel the pulsations between the tendons in the center of your wrist bone directly down from your thumb.
- Neck: Place two fingers at the front center of your throat. Move one to two inches to the left or right and feel your carotid pulse. Press lightly on only one side of your neck at a time. Count your pulse for 10 seconds; start the count at zero. Multiply this number by six to determine your resting heart rate (beats per minute).

Practice taking your pulse so it is easier for you to find after exercise. Check your heart rate after warm-up exercises, after each five to ten minutes of aerobic exercise, and after your cooldown exercises. (If you participate in an outpatient cardiac rehabilitation program, this information can help you evaluate your progress.) When your heart rate drops 20 to 40 beats in the first minute after you stop, you'll know that you're in fabulous shape!

Aerobic versus Anaerobic . . . What's the Difference?

AEROBIC EXERCISE	ANAEROBIC EXERCISE
A physical activity that uses the same large muscle group rhythmically for a period of 15 to 20 minutes (or longer) while you maintain 60 to 80 percent of your maximum heart rate.	Exercise that, no matter how strenuous, does not cause increases in respiration and heart rate. For example, many forms of weight training work the muscles, but not the heart and lungs.
Trains the heart, lungs, and cardiovascular system to process and deliver oxygen more quickly and efficiently to every part of the body.	Draws energy from carbohydrates that are stored in your muscles for short bursts of activity (i.e., sprinting, jumping, lifting heavy weights, activities of daily living).
Involves increased breathing and elevated heart rate over an extended period of time. Affected by frequency, duration, and intensity of activity. Aerobic activity is long in duration yet low in intensity.	Involves short, intensive activities lasting less than 60 seconds or longer activities that are intermittent (i.e., boxing, football) that consist of repeated high-intensity bouts of activity.
Frequency = how often you perform aerobic activity	Does not burn fat, but bigger muscles burn more calories. Essential for strength building and muscle gain.
Duration = the time spent at each session	Example: Push-ups, stomach crunches, pull-ups, lifting weights (high in intensity but relatively short in duration)
Intensity = the percentage of your maximum heart rate at which you work	
Burns fat, tones muscles, and increases lean body mass, reduces fatigue and increases energy levels.	
Examples: walking, bicycling, jogging, swimming, aerobic classes, cross-country skiing (low in intensity but long in duration)	

WHAT ACTIVITIES BURN THE MOST CALORIES?

The amount of calories you burn during exercise varies depending on your age, sex, weight, and metabolism, as well as how intensely you perform the exercise. However, some physical activities do burn more calories than others. Below are lists of activities, categorized by the average number of calories burned in twelve minutes.

BEST CALORIE BURNERS	
ACTIVITY	CALORIES BURNED
Running (8-minute mile)	168
Karate (tae kwon do)	154
Circuit weight training	151
Cycling (15 mph)	142
Downhill skiing	140
Swimming, vigorous	136
Jogging (10-minute mile)	132
Spinning class (indoor cycling)	125
In-line skating	120
GOOD CALORIE BURNERS	
ACTIVITY	CALORIES BURNED
Cycling (12 mph)	114
Soccer	114
Jumping rope (60–80 skips/minute)	114
Ski machine	113
Swimming (freestyle, 50 yards/minute)	105
Aerobic dance	103

Activity	Calories burned
Swimming (freestyle, 35 yards/minute)	99
Tennis (singles)	93
Gardening (digging)	92
Racquetball	91
Ice/roller-skating	90
Horseback riding	86
Skiing (water, downhill, cross-country)	84
Rowing machine	83
Walking (15-minute mile, hills)	82
Scrubbing floors, mowing grass (push)	80
Badminton	78
Gardening	77
Golf (carry clubs)	72
Volleyball	68
Hiking	67
Walking (20-minute mile, hills)	65
Kayaking, Ping-Pong	60
Walking (15-minute mile, flat)	58
Water aerobics	56
Raking leaves	54
Walking (20-minute mile, flat)	48
Dancing (social)	42
Bowling	18

Fill Up to Slim Down Exercise Prescription 2: Strength Training

According to the ACSM, strength training should be an integral part of every adult's fitness program. Lifting weights or using circuit-training equipment improves body shape and tone, boosts metabolic rate, and increases lean muscle tissue.

As you get older, strength training becomes even more important. According to the ACSM, loss of muscle mass (sarcopenia) begins after age thirty and is accompanied by reduced muscle density and increased fat between the muscles. Muscle atrophy is directly proportional to age-related decreases in strength.

The ACSM suggests conditioning all major muscle groups two to three times a week. If possible, consult a certified exercise professional, such as a personal trainer, to instruct you on how to begin. Certified trainers work at fitness centers and gyms, and many centers provide exercise instruction to new members.

If you plan to do strength training at home, invest in an illustrated book geared to beginners—learning how to do the movements correctly will help you avoid injury. But in general, here are some top tips for strength-training success.

- *Warm up and cool down* before and after workouts.
- *Stretch* before and after workouts, too.
- *Think big to small.* Move from bigger muscles (legs, chest, upper back) to smaller muscles (shoulders, arms, abdominals).
- *Start small.* Start with weights you can lift comfortably. You should be able to do 8 to 12 repetitions without sacrificing form. Start at one set, and work up to two or three sets.
- *Focus on posture and form.* Tighten abdominal muscles, stand tall, and don't arch your back.

- *Work opposing muscles at each session.* Each muscle group has an opposing one with which it works, so it is important to work both—for example, the quadriceps and hamstrings (on the front and back of the thigh), or the biceps and triceps (on the front and back of the upper arm). An imbalance between opposing muscles increases the risk of injury.
- *Go through the motion.* Lift and lower the weight in a full range of motion. Don't lock your joints. Use slow and controlled movements.
- *Slow it down.* Count two to four seconds as you lift and another two to four as you lower. Make the muscles do the work, not the force of your movement!
- *Breathe through the motion.* Exhale during exertion to prevent feelings of faintness or lightheadedness.
- *Use* enough resistance to fatigue muscles without strain.
- *Never* sacrifice form for number of repetitions (if you can't perform the last one as efficiently as the first, lower your weight).
- *Increase* weights by no more than 5 percent at a time.
- *Give yourself a day to recover!* Don't work the same muscle groups two days in a row. Your muscles get stronger when they're worked and then repaired.
- *Sore is okay; pain is not!* Listen to your body. If something hurts, stop. Take a few days off to rest the muscle and then start again with light resistance.

BURN, BABY, BURN!

Good news—you burn calories even while you do the dishes, vacuum, and sweep. Here's the amount of calories you'll burn in twelve minutes performing the chores below.

ACTIVITY	CALORIES BURNED
Wash windows	50
Wash/polish car	45
Mopping	44
Sweeping	44
Grocery shopping	35
Vacuuming	35
Painting	27
Washing dishes	24
Making beds	18

Fill Up to Slim Down Exercise Prescription 3: Stretching

As we age, our muscles, tendons, and ligaments start to shorten, tighten, and lose their elasticity. Over time, this can restrict our movement, as well as our ability to exercise. Taking a few short minutes to stretch regularly, including before and after workouts, can help safeguard your flexibility. Research shows that the longer you hold a stretch, the more the muscle will stretch. Stretching also can help prevent injury and help lessen the severity of an injury.

When you stretch, you lengthen your muscles and tendons. When a muscle is flexible, it enables the joint to completely flex, extend, and move in multiple directions (known as range of motion). Other benefits of regular stretching include reduced stiffness and pain, balanced muscle groups, improved posture, reduced risk of low back pain, increased blood and nutrient flow to tissues, and enhanced pleasure in physical activities. Flexibility stretches should be performed daily.

Stretch for ten to fifteen minutes before every workout to relax your body, improve your coordination, warm your muscles, and reduce the risk of injury. Stretch all the major muscle groups. Don't bounce, and don't hold your breath as you stretch. Hold each stretch from forty to sixty seconds, maintaining continuous tension on the muscle. You should not feel pain. Exhale as you stretch, allowing your muscles to relax.

Perform the same stretches after your workout, too. It helps your body cool down, returns your heartbeat to pre-workout rate, and helps relieve tired muscles.

 FIVE TIPS FOR SURE SUCCESS

1. *Make sure you're fit to get fit.* Consult your doctor before you begin any exercise program, especially if you have heart trouble, undiagnosed chest pains, diabetes, high blood pressure, arthritis or other bone or joint problems, often feel faint or dizzy, or are or might be pregnant.
2. *Warm up.* Before you begin a workout (including stretching), warm up your muscles. You can march in place, do light calisthenics, or gently go through the motions of the exercise you will be performing.
3. *Cool it.* "Cool down" after a workout by walking slowly (or slowing the pace of the exercise) until your heartbeat is ten to fifteen beats above its resting rate. The purpose of cooling down is to bring the heart rate down to its normal rate and to get the blood circulating freely back to the heart. Do not stop exercise suddenly; this could cause you to faint or place undue stress on your heart.

(continued)

4. *S-T-R-E-T-C-H!* Finish each workout session with slow stretches. Stretching maintains overall flexibility while it reduces the risk of injury and muscle soreness.

5. *Drink up.* Drink two eight-ounce cups of water about two hours before exercise, another cup every twenty minutes during exercise, and one to two cups within thirty minutes after your workout.

Exercise Fact and Fiction

Does lifting weights "bulk up" a woman's body? Does muscle turn to fat when you stop working out? Don't let the exercise myths below stand in the way of fitness! Here are some of the most common myths about exercise, as well as the facts.

Fiction #1: Exercise makes you lose weight.
Fact: No matter how you cut it, calories do matter: Before you can lose weight, you have to burn more calories than you take in. The Fill Up to Slim Down way of eating fills you up, yet teaches your body to be satisfied with fewer calories. It also diminishes the cravings for fatty, sugary food that so often plague dieters. So on the Fill Up to Slim Down plan, you eat more while you lose more!

Fiction #2: If you don't have (at least) twenty minutes to exercise, skip it. Same goes for weight lifting—without three full sets, it's not worth the effort.
Fact: Nothin' could be wronger than to think you must go longer! Any exercise is better than none. You get the same benefits from three ten-minute aerobic sessions as you do from one thirty-minute session; push your muscles to fatigue and one set will build strength.

Fiction #3: Strength training makes women "bulky."
Fact: Compared to men, women have less of the male sex hormone testosterone, which is the key to developing large muscles. Strength training two or three times a week, doing a variety of exercises for the major muscle groups, will create a lean and toned appearance, rather than bulky muscles.

Fiction #4: Exercise should focus on duration rather than intensity.
Fact: The harder you push, the more you'll burn, and the more weight you'll ultimately lose. Of course, don't push harder than your body can go—proceed at a challenging yet comfortable pace.

Fiction #5: If you stop working out, muscle will turn into fat.
Fact: Muscle and fat are completely different tissues. You may *feel* flabbier if you stop exercising, because muscle tissue shrink. Also, when muscles get smaller, they do not require as many calories, so your metabolism slows. So if you eat the same amount of calories, you may gain body fat.

Putting It All Together

Check out the fitness profiles below, find your fitness level, and use the advice to create a safe, effective exercise program. If you've been completely inactive, consult your doctor before you begin any fitness program. Also, regardless of your fitness level, progress at your own pace and listen to your body.

How often do you exercise?	What level is best for you?	Aerobic Activity	Strength Training	Guides
Never or Rarely	Level 1	3 times per week, 20–30 minutes	2 times per week; 20- to 30-minute sessions; work all muscle groups; 1 set = 8–12 reps; skip a day between to allow 24-hour recovery.	Personal trainer, strength training videotapes, books on training methods.
Less than 2 hours per week	Level 2	4 times per week; 30-minute sessions; every other day, increase duration by 1 minute. If too tired later in the day, subtract 1 minute and stick to that for 1 week, then work up in 1-minute increments.	3 times per week; 20- to 30-minute sessions; increase sets from 1–2 (or 2–3) of 12–15 reps/set; if you can't fit in all muscle groups, alternate upper body/trunk one day and lower body the next; *don't* work the same muscle group two days in a row (allow 24-hour recovery).	Same as above.
2 or more hours per week	Level 3	4–5 times per week; increase intensity and duration of workouts to at least 30- to 45-minute sessions; cross train to avoid overuse injuries and to get the best benefits to body.	4+ days per week; 20- to 30-minute sessions; 2–3 sets with 8–12 repetitions per set; complete at least 8 reps body/trunk 1 day and lower body the next.	If your focus is on endurance and toning, use less weight with more repetitions (12–15 per set); if your focus is on strength, use heavier weights and fewer repetitions (8 per set); if you cannot complete at least 8 reps per set, reduce the weight rather than compromise proper form and risk injury.

7   Reduce Stress to Eat Right

It's what you've been waiting for—a diet designed to help you cope with stress. Ready?

BREAKFAST
½ grapefruit
1 slice whole-wheat toast, dry
8 ounces skim milk

LUNCH
4 ounces broiled chicken breast
1 cup steamed spinach
1 cup herb tea
1 Oreo

Mid-Afternoon Snack
Rest of the Oreos in the package
1 pint Rocky Road ice cream

Dinner
1 large pepperoni pizza
½ bag potato chips
4 cans beer
1 Milky Way bar

This is a joke, of course—it's been widely circulated on the Internet. However, it certainly has the ring of truth, doesn't it? How many times have you come home, drained, from a stressful day at work and turned to a pint of ice cream or a bag of chips to make yourself feel better?

Eating in response to stress is your body's way of trying to calm itself. If you're like many people who "stress eat," you may even have develop a preference for foods rich in salt, fat, and sugar (can you say, "comfort foods"?). If overeating is your usual approach to dealing with stress, it's time to develop smarter solutions. Like smoking or heavy drinking—behaviors many people depend on to wind down from stress—overeating to relieve stress is unhealthy, both for your body and your mind, especially if you put yourself down for gaining weight.

This chapter can help you learn how to manage stress so that it doesn't derail your new, healthier way of eating. Remember, it's far better to nourish your soul with relaxation, pleasure, and rest than to overburden your body with sugar and fat, which will add extra pounds to your body—and stress to your mind. But to fight the enemy, you first have to know what you're up against.

HOW STRESSED ARE YOU?

Check out this list of stress producers, and you'll quickly see how fast the stress in your life can add up.

- Life conditions (marriage, separation, or divorce; pregnancy or new baby; promotion or dismissal at work; retirement; new school)
- Worry about money, family, relationships, work, health
- Living conditions (move to new residence, visitors, remodeling)
- Personal habits (diet, exercise, sleep, medication, drugs, alcohol, smoking, caffeine)
- Environment (climate, altitude)
- Illness (self, child, spouse, parent, etc.)
- Death of spouse, family member, or friend
- Working too hard; partying late; compulsive exercise; excessive commitments; troubles with children, in-laws, parents, or boss
- Allergies

This Is Your Appetite on Stress

Stress is the body's response to any demand or pressure. These demands, called stressors, include major life events—marriage, divorce, retirement, the birth of a child—as well as daily or occasional strains, like a long commute or a troubled relationship.

Some stress is beneficial to our lives. Good stress, or "eustress," as researchers call it, can sharpen your thinking and give you an edge that pushes you to give your all. But stress that drags on week after week, month after month puts you at increased risk for heart disease, stroke, diabetes, colds and flu, headaches, digestive problems, and sleep disturbances.

Stress may be accompanied by fatigue, a run-down feeling, forgetfulness, low productivity, or anger or irritation. It can change your eating habits, too. While some people eat less under stress, many people turn to food for comfort.

Stress may even trigger powerful cravings. When you experience a stressful situation or event, your body goes into "fight or flight" mode—a physiological state in which it prepares to either fight or run away from the perceived threat. For example, your heart rate and respiration increase, your pupils dilate (the better to see the threat), and your muscles tighten. Your body also releases the stress hormones adrenaline and cortisol, which help the body mobilize carbohydrates and fat for quick energy. When the stress is over, cortisol acts to increase appetite, urging us to replace the carbohydrates and fat that we used while fleeing or fighting.

There's just one problem: We don't often fight or flee under stress. Instead, we simmer and worry and fret, which doesn't require all that many calories. So we don't need that extra fuel—the doughnut, Doritos, candy bar—because we didn't expend any energy. What happens when you give in to your cravings each time you're stressed out? That's right—most likely, you'll gain weight.

While there's not much you can do to remove stress from your life, you *can* learn to change your reaction to it. You can make wise food choices (which can help give you the energy to fight stress), get back in touch with your body, and try some very basic distressing techniques. Read on to find out how.

STRESSED? PUT DOWN THAT MUG

Can't function without your morning cup of coffee (or three)? Can't do without that mid-afternoon double latte? If you're a java junkie, caffeine may well be compounding your stress.

Found in coffee, chocolate, and many sodas (especially colas), caffeine is a stimulant. If you drink too much of it, or if you're sensitive to caffeine, you may experience an increase in heart rate, blood pressure, and levels of stress hormones.

Caffeine may also magnify your perception of stress. In fact, a study conducted at Duke University Medical Center in Durham, North Carolina, shows that caffeine taken in the morning amplifies stress consistently throughout the day. Put another way, caffeine enhances the effects of everyday stresses, so if you have a stressful job, drinking coffee makes your body respond more to the ordinary stresses you experience.

Ready to cut back? Try these tips.

- To avoid symptoms of caffeine withdrawal, slowly cut back to one to two "cups" (5 ounces each) of coffee per day
- Be aware of hidden caffeine in chocolate, sodas, and medications
- Explore the many alternatives to caffeinated drinks, such as caffeine-free herbal teas and sodas, and that elixir of life, water, iced, with a squeeze of lemon or lime
- To boost your energy without caffeine, take a brisk ten- or fifteen-minute walk

De-Stress with Good Nutrition

Do you skip meals because you "don't have time" to eat? Do you guzzle coffee or caffeinated sodas to keep you going? When you eat under stress, do you tend to choose foods laden with simple sugars and/or fat?

If so, stress may be affecting your diet, and therefore your weight. The tips below can help you make sure you get the healthy foods that can help defuse stress and stress-related food cravings.

Don't skip meals. You rush out the door in the morning, work through lunch or dinner. But your body will make sure you make up for those missed meals, often with a binge. If you take the time to sit down and eat real meals, your blood sugar will stay steady, keeping binges and cravings at bay. Taking the time to eat nourishing meals also gives you the energy and clarity of thought to handle stress in healthy ways, like taking a walk outside rather than to the vending machine.

Reach for "star carbs." By now, you know that complex carbohydrates, which form the core of the Fill Up to Slim Down way of eating, can increase the levels of calming serotonin in your brain—in as little as thirty minutes. Some of these star carbs include fruits and vegetables and whole-grain breads, cereals, and pasta. Try choosing extra-crunchy fruits and vegetables, like apples or baby carrots—all that munching can really take the edge off stress. Or enjoy a serving of salt-free, air-popped popcorn. To make Jyl's "buttered popcorn," spray hot, air-popped popcorn (right out of the popper) with butter-flavored cooking spray. Mix quickly, shake on Butter Buds, then mix again.

Fight "PM Stress" with calcium. Some researchers believe that the fatigue, anxiety, depression, and personality changes of PMS (Premenstrual Syndrome) could be the result of low calcium levels (hypocalcemia). Getting more calcium to minimize PMS is killing two birds with one stone—relief from the weepiness or irritation, and preventing osteoporosis down the road. Aim to eat three calcium-rich foods a day. Low-fat dairy foods such as skim milk, soy, and reduced-fat yogurt are your best bets. If you don't do milk, try a glass of soy milk, calcium-fortified orange juice, salmon, almonds, or broccoli, which are also high in calcium.

Ride out a craving. When you're seized by a stress-related craving for a sugary, fatty food, try riding it out for a few minutes before you give in. This is called "urge-surfing." Like a wave, the intensity of the urge will crest, then break. It may "break" in five, ten, or twenty minutes, but it will break. While you wait, distract yourself—remove old nail polish, do your online banking, or hop on your treadmill or stationary bicycle.

Practice good "eating hygiene." We're not talking about manners, but about eating mindfully. Eat only when you are sitting down, and when you are not doing another activity, such as reading or watching TV. If you eat while you're doing something else, you may eat more than you intended. When you focus on what you're eating, you will be more likely to eat according to your hunger.

Free Yourself from the Stress of a Negative Body Image

Ever felt disconnected from the person you see in the mirror? Ever glimpsed yourself in a store window and wondered, "Is that body really mine?" These feelings aren't unusual in people who have struggled with their weight. Somehow, somewhere, you stop seeing yourself as you are. You may freeze an image of yourself from a fitter time, so you think you look better than you do, or you develop such an antipathy for your reflection that you see yourself as far heavier and more unattractive than you are.

When you can't really "see" what you look like, it's difficult to maintain a healthy body image—or a healthy body. Here are some ways you might begin to get back in touch with your physical self.

Appreciate the machinery. Flawed as it might be, your body is a living, breathing miracle. Take a few minutes each day to marvel at your body's operation, as with each inhalation your hearbeats, your blood pumps, your brain calculates or philosophizes, and your senses experience the world around you. Your legs take you where you want to go; your arms heft heavy sacks of groceries or a child; maybe your abdomen once nourished the child you hold (or once held) in your arms. Find the 90 percent that's good, rather than the 10 percent that you don't like.

Indulge your body. More often than not, a disliked body is a neglected body. If you've been ignoring yours lately, do something nice for it. Treat it to a luxurious scented skin cream. Get a pedicure. Heck, book a session at a nice day spa, or hire a personal trainer for a one-on-one workout session. No matter how big or small the indulgence, it will help you reconnect with your body and provide a respite from the stresses of the day.

Splurge on a massage. There's nothing like a massage to reawaken a body to sensual satisfaction that has nothing to do with sex and everything to do with animal pleasure. If you've never had one, ask friends for recommendations or speak to a therapist at your gym. Start small if you're unsure—book a half hour instead of an hour, ask for a Swedish or sports massage, and remain fully or partially clothed if you're uncomfortable with nudity. Don't be surprised if you feel emotional during a massage. This kind of touch can also free feelings that have been bottled up inside, and becoming aware of them is the first step to finding more peace of mind.

Move your body in new ways. Take yoga, join a cycling class, or add a recreational swim class to your workout schedule. Use your workouts to increase your awareness of how your body feels as it moves and breathes. The better you get to know your body, the better it will start to look and feel and the more you will enjoy your workouts.

Anti-Stress Strategies That Work— Every Time

Get moving. Regular, moderate physical activity may be the best approach to managing stress. Exercise causes the brain to release endorphins, opiumlike substances that produce feelings of euphoria. It also encourages the brain to secrete other chemicals, such as serotonin, dopamine, and norepinephrine, which improve general mood. For more information on exercise, see chapter 6.

Breathe. Not just your average inhale-exhale, breathe-in-blow-out rhythm from your chest. Deep breathing is a method of relaxation that removes tension from your body, and you can do it virtually anywhere. Try this: Sit in a comfortable chair or lie on the floor with a pillow under the small of your back. Breathe in slowly and deeply, pushing your stomach out as you inhale, silently saying "relax" as you exhale. Repeat ten times. Repeat as often as you need to.

Be nice to yourself. Self-put-downs hurt as much as those inflicted by others, maybe even more so. Talk to yourself the way you would talk to others. Would you ever tell your child or friend, "You're a fat slob," or, "You're pathetic—you screwed up your eating again." We didn't think so!

Confide in others. Seek out a good friend, support group, counselor, pastor, rabbi, or other clergy person who listens (without interruption or pushing advice). Experience the freedom to share your feelings and lighten the load. Talking it out clarifies the problem and helps you seek positive solutions.

Learn to say "no." Prioritize your obligations, divide them into piles, and label them: "must-dos," "should-dos," "want-to-dos." Set the piles in front of you so you can see what you're dealing with. Then cut each pile in half. If you just can't say the n-word, try delegating or swapping services with a family member or friend.

Learn a relaxation technique. Deep breathing, yoga, and meditation are just a few of the relaxation techniques that can help you calm down during stressful times. You'll find plenty of books and videos that can help teach you the basics.

Keep a food diary. Writing down everything you eat each day can help you think about what you are eating. You may also note what events are stressful to you and are causing you to eat. For more on keeping a food diary, see chapter 5.

Accept what you can't change. Next time you're in full panic mode, ask yourself, "Is there anything I can do to change this situation?" If not, just accept it (breathe deep!) and move on.

8 Improving Your Heart Health on the Fill Up to Slim Down Diet

Imagine if you could consult your heart before each meal. If you asked it whether it would prefer a burger and fries or a spinach salad and a bowl of hearty lentil soup, you'd get the same answer every time. Your heart is wired for survival, and the salad and lentil soup promise longer life.

Your heart loves foods that are high in fiber and complex carbohydrates, rich in vitamins and minerals, generally low in fat, and found in nature, rather than from boxes, bags, and take-out containers. There are mountains of scientific studies that link a healthy diet to heart health. Here's just a sampling of the findings:

- Substances in soy foods, called isoflavones, can reduce "bad" LDL cholesterol, reducing the risk of heart disease.
- Plant foods are rich in heart-loving plant chemicals, such as quercetin, flavonoids, and polyphenols. These substances may

help prevent blockages in the arteries that supply the heart with blood.

- In both men and women, whole grains lower the risk of heart disease and levels of total and LDL cholesterol.

Score another point for the Fill Up to Slim Down way of eating! By designing meals around foods that offer more satisfaction for fewer calories, you can eat enough to feel full, achieve maximum nutrient value, lose excess weight, and contribute to heart health. Let's turn our attention to one crucial substance found in the Fill Up to Slim Down plan that can help you achieve all of these goals.

Fiber: the Heart of a Healthy Diet

Found only in plant foods, fiber is a special type of carbohydrate that passes through the digestive system intact, without being broken down into nutrients. Despite overwhelming evidence that a diet rich in fiber helps protect cardiovascular health, we're not eating enough of it. We consume only a tenth of the fiber that we did a century ago. While it's recommended that adults consume from 20 to 35 grams each day, studies have shown that the average American adult consumes only 7 to 15 grams. So fiber up your diet, and your heart will thank you.

There are two types of dietary fiber—soluble and insoluble. Your diet should include both, because each helps you improve or maintain your health in a different way.

By including *soluble fiber* in your diet, you may be able to lower the level of plaque-forming LDL ("bad") cholesterol in your blood. As soluble fiber passes through your gastrointestinal tract, it binds to bile acids and carries them through the intestines.

A diet high in soluble fiber can help you protect your heart. A 1999 study of U.S. women published in the *Journal of the American Medical Association* found that a diet high in soluble fiber, particularly breakfast cereals, can reduce a woman's risk of heart disease up to 23 percent. Soluble fiber also helps to promote regularity, which can protect against diverticular disease, irritable bowel syndrome (IBS), and gallstones.

The best sources of soluble fiber include:

- Legumes, beans, and peas
- Nuts and seeds
- Oat bran and other types of bran
- Apples, oranges, and pears
- Carrots, potatoes, and squash
- Corn and popcorn

Insoluble fiber is indigestible and increases bulk in the intestines as it absorbs water. Bulk helps to maintain the proper functioning of the intestines by keeping bowels regular and, in turn, preventing constipation. Because insoluble fiber speeds the movement of potentially carcinogenic substances through the digestive system, it also helps to reduce your risk of colon and colorectal cancer. In addition, by softening stools, insoluble fiber may help to prevent hemorrhoids and diverticular disease.

The best sources of insoluble fiber include:

- Wheat bran and whole-grain products such as bread, crackers, some breakfast cereals, bran muffins
- Brown rice, kidney beans
- Skins of many fruits, such as pears, apples, and prunes
- Vegetables including green beans, broccoli, peppers, spinach, carrots, tomatoes, and artichokes (these may also contain some soluble fiber)
- Almonds, Brazil nuts, chunky peanut butter
- Popcorn

Tackling Your Risk Factors

The Arizona Heart Institute (http://www.azheart.com) offers an inter-
active test to determine cardiac risk, which is based on the most current
studies. I encourage my patients to take an active role in their heart
health, and I want my readers to know the facts and take positive action,
too. Read on to learn the five biggest threats to your heart—and, more
important, what you can do to reduce them. It should be no surprise that
the Fill Up to Slim Down way of eating can play a vital role in preventing heart disease, or managing it if you've already been diagnosed with it.

 FOUR CALL-THE-DOCTOR SYMPTOMS

Heart disease is the number-one cause of death in the United States, and
contrary to what many think, it isn't just a man's disease. In fact, it's the
leading cause of death for American women. If you have any of the symptoms below, call your health-care provider immediately.

- **Chest pain.** Pain, tightness, or pressure in your chest can occur
  when your heart doesn't get enough oxygen. Angina that occurs
  with exercise is called stable angina, while unstable angina occurs
  unexpectedly or when you're at rest. Unstable angina is the more
  serious of the two and could signal an impending heart attack.
- **Shortness of breath.** This may be a sign that your heart is having
  trouble pumping blood around your body. The resulting buildup
  of fluid in and around your lungs can make it hard to breathe.
- **Swelling in the legs and feet.** It's not always caused by heart disease, but holding fluid in your legs can be a warning sign, especially if you have other symptoms, such as shortness of breath.
- **Calf pain when you walk.** This condition, called claudication, occurs when your muscles are not getting enough oxygen because of
  blocked arteries. Blockages in the leg arteries may mean there are
  blockages in the coronary arteries as well.

RISK FACTOR 1: HIGH CHOLESTEROL

There are two kinds of cholesterol: dietary cholesterol, the kind in food, and blood cholesterol, a fatlike substance in the blood. Your body makes some cholesterol naturally. But when there's too much of it in your blood, the excess builds up on the walls of the arteries that carry blood to the heart. This buildup is called atherosclerosis, commonly called hardening of the arteries. Atherosclerosis narrows the arteries and can slow or block blood flow to the heart. If your heart can't get enough blood and oxygen, you may experience chest pain. If the blood supply is completely blocked, the result is a heart attack.

You can't *feel* high cholesterol, so you won't know if it's too high unless you have it checked. That's important, because the sooner you know that it's too high, the sooner you can lower it—and reduce your risk of developing heart disease.

The latest studies seem to indicate that when it comes to blood cholesterol, the lower the number, the better. Here are the current guidelines for total cholesterol, according to the National Institutes of Health. (By the way, cholesterol levels are measured in milligrams per deciliter of blood, or mg/dL.)

Total cholesterol of less than 200 mg/dL: Desirable
Total cholesterol of 200–239 mg/dL: Borderline High
Total cholesterol of 240 mg/dL and above: High

Take Action Now!
If you haven't had your cholesterol checked within the past year, ask your doctor to write you a prescription. It's a simple test, and you can go to any medical testing facility to have blood drawn and analyzed.

If the number is higher than your doctor would like, he's likely to recommend lifestyle changes, such as healthy eating and regular physical activity. Both can help you lose weight—a major risk factor for heart disease—and lower your cholesterol. (Check with your doctor before you start any exercise program, especially if you've been inactive for a long time.) If lifestyle factors don't bring about enough of a change, your doctor may prescribe medication.

Heart-smart tip: Eat your spinach! It's an excellent source of folate, which has been shown to lower blood levels of homocysteine, an amino acid linked to heart disease. In one study, women who consumed the most of this B vitamin were 31 percent less likely to die of heart disease than those who consumed the least. Other good sources of folate include legumes, fortified cereals, and Brussels sprouts.

RISK FACTOR 2: LOW "GOOD CHOLESTEROL," HIGH "BAD CHOLESTEROL"

Your total cholesterol doesn't tell the entire story—your high-density lipoprotein (HDL) cholesterol and low-density lipoprotein (LDL) cholesterol also figure into the equation. Research has linked high HDL levels to a reduced risk of heart disease, and lower LDL and triglycerides to a reduced risk of heart attack, stroke, and death.

Why is HDL cholesterol the good guy? Because it picks up fragments of cholesterol and transports them to the liver for repackaging or disposal. The bad guy, LDL, is the main source of cholesterol buildup and blockage in the arteries.

You'll also want to check your levels of triglycerides—fatty deposits in blood that also raise heart disease risk. Triglyceride levels that are borderline high (150–199 mg/dL) or high (200 mg/dL or more) indicate increased risk. Bear in mind, though, that studies have demonstrated that people who have suffered heart attacks can have normal HDL and LDL numbers.

CHOLESTEROL BY THE NUMBERS

If you're twenty and over, you should have your cholesterol measured at least once every five years. The best test? A "lipoprotein profile," which measures total cholesterol, LDL and HDL cholesterol, and triglycerides. How do *your* numbers compare to the tables below?

TOTAL CHOLESTEROL	CATEGORY
Less than 200 mg/dL	Desirable
200–239 mg/dL	Borderline high
240 mg/dL and above	High

LDL CHOLESTEROL	CATEGORY
Less than 100 mg/dL	Optimal
100–129 mg/dL	Near optimal/above optimal
130–159 mg/dL	Borderline high
160–189 mg/dL	High
190 mg/dL and above	Very high

Take Action Now!

An HDL level under 40 is a major risk factor for heart disease, whereas an HDL level of 60 or above is normal. Your goal is to increase your HDL levels to 40 to 50 mg/dL or more, and your LDL levels to less than 100 mg/dL. Following the Fill Up to Slim Down program—including the exercise component—can help. If lifestyle changes don't work, or if you have additional risk factors, your doctor may prescribe medication.

Heart-smart tip: Consider adding tofu and other soy foods to your Fill Up to Slim Down meals two or three times a week. Research suggests that soy may help protect the heart and arteries by making the fats in blood less damaging and discouraging the buildup of plaque in the arteries.

RISK FACTOR 3: SMOKING

Is anyone out there still smoking? Unfortunately, the answer is yes. While many cities and states have enacted laws to limit smoking in public places, millions of people still smoke, and new smokers join their ranks every day.

Most smokers—maybe even you?—may not have given a thought to smoking's effect on the heart. But the facts are undeniable: One in five deaths from cardiovascular diseases is attributable to smoking.

Take Action Now!

Give up smoking, and you reduce your risk factors almost immediately.

If you've tried to quit before and not succeeded, keep trying. You may find that a combination of different strategies is the way to go, from using an over-the-counter aid to attending regular stress-reduction classes, including yoga. Reducing dependence on nicotine will lower your risk, and eliminating it will have far-reaching medical benefits.

Heart-smart tip: Whether you're a current or ex-smoker, make a point of eating citrus fruits, including tangerines. An international team of researchers reported that beta-cryptoxanthin, a substance from the carotenoid family of plant chemicals, reduced lung cancer by more than 30 percent for those whose diets provided the highest amount. Citrus fruits are rich in beta-cryptoxanthin, which previous research has suggested may promote the health of the respiratory tract. Of course, if you're a current smoker, your best bet is to quit.

A WORD ABOUT ALCOHOL

Over the past few years, the health benefits of moderate drinking have been widely reported. Population studies in several countries have reported that "light to moderate alcohol consumption" appears to be linked to a reduction in mortality from cardiovascular disease. "Moderate" consumption is defined as one drink per day for women and two per day for men. (One drink equals 12 ounces of beer, 5 ounces of wine, or 1.5 ounces of distilled spirits.)

It may be that the benefits of alcohol are on the blood vessels and help prevent blockages in the arteries to the heart and brain. This might be related to alcohol's effect on "good" HDL cholesterol. Moderate amounts of alcohol may also act as a blood thinner, lowering the risk of heart attack, and improve the body's sensitivity to insulin, helping to prevent diabetes.

Does this mean that if you don't drink, you should start? No. Because the degree of risk reduction is small and because we know that moderate to heavy alcohol consumption can have a harmful effect, no one is recommending that non-drinkers pick up the habit. For example, there is evidence that breast cancer rates are higher among women who drink moderately. If you have a history of breast cancer in your family, ask your doctor about whether you should drink alcohol.

Remember, too, that drinking and weight loss don't go hand in hand. Not only is alcohol fairly high in calories with little or no nutrition, it also loosens your inhibitions. In other words, it may encourage you to eat things you shouldn't—like Buffalo wings, gooey nachos, or calorie-laden desserts.

RISK FACTOR 4: HIGH BLOOD PRESSURE

High blood pressure—when blood pressure stays elevated over time—makes the heart work too hard and contributes to hardening of the arteries. People with high blood pressure are three times more likely to develop coronary heart disease, six times more likely to develop congestive heart failure, and seven times more likely to have a stroke.

A blood pressure level of 140/90 mmHg or higher is considered high.

A level between 120/80 mmHg and 139/89 mmHg indicates a condition called prehypertension. People with this condition don't have high blood pressure yet, but are likely to develop it in the future.

Take Action Now!

Get your blood pressure checked, of course. But not with home testing devices or at the pharmacy or mall—they aren't always accurate. Have your doctor do it. Generally speaking, doctors diagnose high blood pressure on the basis of two or more readings, taken on several occasions. Combining the Fill Up to Slim Down way of eating with other lifestyle changes like losing weight through a healthy diet, regular exercise, and reducing your stress level can help bring it down. If lifestyle changes alone are not effective in keeping your pressure controlled, your doctor may prescribe blood pressure medications.

Heart-smart tip: DASH to the Web site of the American Dietetic Association to learn about a diet called Dietary Approaches to Stop Hypertension. In a large, government-funded study of individuals with moderate hypertension, it was found that a low-fat diet high in fruits and vegetables and low-fat dairy foods can lower their blood pressure as much as medication—and in as little as two weeks. To learn more, log on to the Web site: http://www.eatright.org/Public/NutritionInformation/92_nfs0899.cfm.

RISK FACTOR 5: DIABETES

The hormone insulin is necessary for the body to be able to use sugar, the body's main source of energy. In the most common form of diabetes, type 2, either the body does not produce enough insulin or cells ignore it, causing the glucose to build up in the blood. Eventually, high blood glucose levels damage many of the body's vital organs, including the heart.

Heart disease is the leading cause of death in people with diabetes. Research has shown that these two serious medical concerns often show up in the same patients, yet diabetes is another disease with few obvious warning signs. Many cases go undiagnosed for months, even years, and during that time arterial disease in the kidneys, eyes, and peripheral circulation systems manifest themselves.

Take Action Now!

If you have any of the common symptoms of diabetes—tiredness, thirst, frequent urination, blurry vision, or sores that do not heal—see your doctor immediately. However, most people with diabetes have no symptoms, so you'll need to depend on a number of factors to determine your risk. Schedule an appointment if you're overweight, if diabetes runs in your family, if you have given birth to a baby who weighed more than nine pounds at birth, or if you have high blood pressure or high cholesterol.

Heart-smart tip: Get your beans—navy, kidney, pinto, whichever variety you prefer. They're excellent sources of fiber, which has been shown to have a positive effect on diabetes. Moreover, legumes have been shown to balance blood-sugar levels and help the body respond better to insulin. Enjoy whole grains, too. In a large government study of nurses, those who ate the least whole-grain cereal fiber and the most white bread and other refined carbohydrates had more than twice the risk of developing diabetes over six years of follow-up.

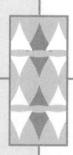

Recipes

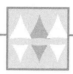

Breakfast

Banana Nut Bread

EASY • DO AHEAD • FREEZE   *Serves: 8*

3 bananas, mashed
½ cup egg substitute
1 teaspoon vanilla extract
½ cup sugar
½ cup brown sugar

1 cup whole-wheat flour
1 cup all-purpose flour
1 teaspoon cinnamon
1 teaspoon baking soda
2 tablespoon chopped walnuts

Preheat the oven to 350 degrees. Spray a 9x5-inch loaf pan with cooking spray. Combine the bananas, egg substitute, vanilla, sugar, and brown sugar in a large bowl; beat with an electric mixer until creamy and smooth. Combine the flours, cinnamon, and baking soda in a zip-top bag; shake well. Gradually add to the banana mixture until all the ingredients are moistened and blended. Fold in the walnuts. Spoon the batter into the loaf pan and bake for 45 to 60 minutes, until a toothpick inserted in the center comes out clean. Cool for 5 minutes before removing from the pan. Slice and serve.

Nutrition per serving: Calories 233 • Fat 1.3g • Carbohydrates 52g • Protein 6g • Cholesterol 0mg • Dietary fiber 3g • Sodium 126mg
Exchanges: 4 other carbs
Carb Choices: 4

Updated federal guidelines state that blood pressure readings of 120 to 139 (systolic) or 80 to 89 (diastolic) put you in a "prehypertension" category and call for lifestyle changes including: weight loss (if needed); increased exercise; maintenance of heart-healthy diet; and reduced salt intake.

Banana Pancakes

EASY • DO AHEAD • FREEZE   *Serves:* 6

1 cup all-purpose flour
½ cup quick-cooking oatmeal,
    uncooked
1 tablespoon baking powder
½ teaspoon cinnamon
1 cup skim milk
½ cup plus 2 tablespoons egg
    substitute

2 large ripe bananas, peeled and
    sliced
1 tablespoon sugar
sugar-free maple-flavored syrup,
    optional

Combine the flour, oatmeal, baking powder, and cinnamon in a large bowl; mix well. Combine the milk and egg substitute in a medium bowl; blend well. Add the milk mixture to the flour mixture all at once and mix until the dry ingredients are moistened. Combine the sliced bananas with the sugar in a small bowl; toss to coat the bananas and set aside. Spray a large nonstick skillet with cooking spray and heat over medium-high heat. Pour the batter ¼ cup at a time; top each pancake with several banana slices. Cook the pancakes until the tops begin to bubble and the edges are lightly browned. Turn the pancakes and cook until lightly browned on the other side. Serve with syrup, if desired.

Nutrition per serving: Calories 175 • Fat 0.9g • Carbohydrates 36g • Protein 6g •
    Cholesterol 1mg • Dietary fiber 2g • Sodium 203mg
Exchanges: 2 starch
Carb Choices: 2

Flavor your morning coffee with nonfat half-and-half and sugar substitutes instead of cream, sugar, and other syrupy additions to specialty coffee drinks—you'll save yourself a whopping 250 to 500 calories.

Berry Breakfast with Crunch Topping

EASY • DO AHEAD   *Serves: 4*

4 medium apples, peeled, cored, and sliced
½ cup blueberries, fresh or frozen
½ cup raspberries, fresh or frozen
1 cup sliced strawberries
¾ cup brown sugar, divided
¼ cup frozen juice concentrate (apple, orange, or pineapple), thawed
¼ cup flour, divided
1½ teaspoons ground cinnamon
1 cup quick-cooking oatmeal, uncooked
3 tablespoons nonfat yogurt (blueberry, strawberry, or vanilla)

Preheat the oven to 350 degrees. Spray an 8-inch square baking dish with cooking spray. Combine the apples, blueberries, raspberries, strawberries, ¼ cup of the brown sugar, juice concentrate, 2 tablespoons of the flour, and cinnamon in a medium bowl; stir until the fruit is coated. Spoon the fruit mixture into the baking dish. Combine the oatmeal, the remaining ½ cup of brown sugar, and 2 tablespoons of flour in a small bowl; mix well. Gradually add the yogurt and mix with your fingertips until the mixture is crumbly. Sprinkle evenly over the fruit mixture. Bake for 30 to 35 minutes, until the fruit is tender and the top is lightly browned. Serve hot or cold.

Nutrition per serving: Calories 397 • Fat 2.1g • Carbohydrates 94g • Protein 5g • Cholesterol <1mg • Dietary fiber 6g • Sodium 26mg
Exchanges: 3 fruit • 2 starch • 1 other carb
Carb Choices: 6

Berries, rich in antioxidants and fiber, may help lower your risk of developing heart disease and certain types of cancer. They are also associated with slowing age-related declines in nerve and brain function.

Breakfast Burrito

EASY   *Serves: 4*

1 cup egg substitute
¼ cup nonfat half-and-half
¼ teaspoon pepper
¾ cup frozen chopped broccoli,
  thawed and drained
¾ cup canned diced tomatoes,
  drained well

4 low-fat whole-wheat flour
  tortillas
1 cup chunky-style salsa
½ cup nonfat sour cream

Combine the egg substitute, half-and-half, pepper, broccoli, and tomatoes in a medium bowl. Mix well. Spray a nonstick skillet with cooking spray and heat over medium-high heat. Pour the egg mixture into the skillet; cook, stirring frequently, until the eggs are cooked through. Remove the skillet from the heat. Wrap the tortillas in damp paper towel; microwave on high heat for 20 to 30 seconds. Spoon the eggs down the center of the tortillas; roll and serve with salsa and sour cream.

Nutrition per serving: Calories 216 • Fat 0.7g • Carbohydrates 37g • Protein 13g •
  Cholesterol 0mg • Dietary fiber 4g • Sodium 991mg
Exchanges: 1 very lean meat • 1 vegetable • 2 starch
Carb Choices: 2

Adding beans to your diet will reduce the risk of disease. Except for wheat bran, no food is more fiber-rich than beans. High in soluble fiber (to lower cholesterol) and folate (lowers homocysteine levels), beans help prevent certain cancers, heart disease, diabetes, and stroke.

Breakfast Muffins with Almond Glaze

EASY • DO AHEAD   *Serves: 12*

¼ cup egg substitute

1 egg white

¾ teaspoon almond extract, divided

¼ cup crushed pineapple; do not drain

⅓ cup applesauce

⅓ cup nonfat vanilla yogurt

½ cup sugar

1½ cups all-purpose flour

1 teaspoon baking powder

¼ cup powdered sugar

1 to 1½ teaspoon skim milk

Preheat the oven to 350 degrees. Spray muffin tin with cooking spray. Combine the egg substitute, egg white, ½ teaspoon of the almond extract, pineapple, applesauce, yogurt, and sugar in a large bowl; mix until smooth and creamy. Add the flour and baking powder; stir the ingredients just until moistened. Fill the muffin cups with batter. Bake for 15 to 20 minutes, until a toothpick inserted in the center comes out clean. Remove the muffins from the pan and cool for 5 minutes. While the muffins are cooling, combine the powdered sugar, the remaining ¼ teaspoon of almond extract, and the skim milk (add enough milk so the glaze can be drizzled over the muffins); drizzle over warm muffins and serve immediately.

Nutrition per serving: Calories 111 • Fat 0.1g • Carbohydrates 25g • Protein 3g • Cholesterol <1mg • Dietary fiber 1g • Sodium 44mg

Exchanges: 2 other carbs

Carb Choices: 2

Seventy-eight percent of people who maintain weight loss for more than five years eat breakfast every day.

Egg and Tortilla Casserole

AVERAGE • DO AHEAD   *Serves: 6*

1 cup canned black beans, drained well	1 cup nonfat sour cream
1 cup chunky-style salsa	1 cup nonfat half-and-half
5 10-inch low-fat flour tortillas, cut into 1-inch strips	½ cup Southwest Egg Beaters
1½ cups nonfat shredded cheddar cheese	2 large egg whites
	¼ teaspoon pepper

Spray a 9x13-inch baking dish with cooking spray. Combine the beans and salsa in a bowl; mix well. Arrange a third of the tortilla strips in the bottom of the baking dish. Top with ½ cup of the cheese. Spoon 1 cup of the bean mixture on top of the cheese; repeat the procedure with a third of the tortilla strips, ½ cup of cheese, 1 cup of the bean mixture, and the remaining tortilla strips. Combine the sour cream, half-and-half, Egg Beaters, egg whites, and pepper in a medium bowl; whisk until frothy. Pour the egg mixture over the tortilla strips; top with the remaining ½ cup of cheese. Cover and refrigerate for at least 6 hours or overnight. Twenty minutes before you are ready to bake, remove the casserole from the refrigerator and let stand at room temperature for 15 to 20 minutes. Preheat the oven to 350 degrees. Cover the casserole with foil and bake for 20 minutes; remove the cover and bake for 15 to 20 minutes, until lightly browned and cooked through.

Nutrition per serving: Calories 261 • Fat 0.5g • Carbohydrates 39g • Protein 20g • Cholesterol 0mg • Dietary fiber 3g • Sodium 1,031mg
Exchanges: 2½ starch • 1 very lean meat • 1 vegetable
Carb Choices: 3

Substitution tip: For each cup of sour cream, substitute half a cup nonfat cottage cheese plus half a cup nonfat plain yogurt blended in a food processor or blender until smooth.

Eggs-traordinary Omelette Florentine

EASY   *Serves: 2*

1 cup frozen chopped spinach,   3 tablespoons nonfat half-
  thawed and drained   and-half
¼ cup frozen diced onions,   ⅛ teaspoon pepper
  thawed and drained   ½ cup nonfat shredded
4 large egg whites   mozzarella cheese
1 cup egg substitute

Spray a nonstick skillet or omelette pan with cooking spray. Preheat the broiler on high heat. Combine the spinach and onions in a medium bowl; microwave on high heat for 3 to 4 minutes, until hot. Combine the egg whites, egg substitute, half-and-half, and pepper in a medium bowl; whisk until completely blended. Turn the stove top on medium-high heat; let the pan get hot for 45 to 60 seconds. Pour the egg mixture into the pan; let the eggs set, carefully lifting several times so the eggs can cook evenly. Spoon the spinach mixture on top; sprinkle with mozzarella cheese. Place the skillet under the broiler; cook for 45 to 60 seconds (watching carefully), just until the cheese is melted. If the skillet has a rubber handle, cover completely with heavy-duty foil.

Nutrition per serving: Calories 121 • Fat 0.2g • Carbohydrates 13g • Protein 32g •
  Cholesterol 0mg • Dietary fiber 2g • Sodium 764mg
Exchanges: 2 vegetable • 2 very lean meat
Carb Choices: 1

Foods with high water or fiber content tend to fill you up faster, according to researchers at Penn State University. The idea is that you'll eat less of (and it'll take longer to eat) a spinach omelette versus a plate of scrambled eggs.

VARIATIONS

Substitute chopped broccoli for spinach. Or substitute nonfat/low-fat cheddar cheese for mozzarella.

Missing certain ingredients? No need to worry . . .

2 egg whites = ¼ cup egg substitute

1 tablespoon half-and-half = 1 tablespoon milk, 1 tablespoon water, or
   1 tablespoon cottage cheese

¼ cup chopped onions = ¼ to ½ teaspoon onion powder

Fiberful Pineapple Zucchini Bread

EASY · DO AHEAD · FREEZE   *Serves: 12*

½ cup crushed pineapple in
   juice; do not drain
¼ cup skim milk
4 large egg whites
¼ cup honey
1 cup all-purpose flour
1¼ cups whole-wheat flour
½ cup wheat germ

¼ cup ground flaxseed
1 teaspoon ground cinnamon
½ teaspoon nutmeg
½ teaspoon baking soda
2 tablespoons baking powder
3 cups shredded zucchini
¾ cup raisins

Preheat the oven to 350 degrees. Spray a 9x5-inch loaf pan with cooking spray. Combine the crushed pineapple with juice, skim milk, egg whites, and honey in a large bowl; mix until blended. Combine the all-purpose flour, whole-wheat flour, wheat germ, ground flaxseed, cinnamon, nutmeg, baking soda, and baking powder in a large zip-top bag; shake vigorously until completely blended. Add the flour mixture to the mixing bowl, blending until ingredients are moistened. Fold in the zucchini and raisins. Spoon the batter into the loaf pan. Bake for 60 to 70 minutes, until a toothpick inserted in the center comes out clean. Cool in the pan for 5 minutes; remove from the pan and cool completely before slicing and serving.

Nutrition per serving: Calories 178 · Fat 1.6g · Carbohydrates 37g · Protein 6g ·
  Cholesterol 0mg · Dietary fiber 4g · Sodium 224mg
Exchanges: 2 other carb
Carb Choices: 2

> The easiest place to start getting the 30 grams of fiber you need every day is at breakfast. Look for a high-fiber whole-grain cereal or bread, which will keep you feeling fuller longer.

French Toast Pockets

EASY · DO AHEAD · FREEZE   *Serves: 6*

12 1-inch thick slices French bread
½ cup nonfat cream cheese, softened
¼ teaspoon orange extract
1 cup egg substitute
4 egg whites
¼ cup nonfat half-and-half
1 teaspoon cinnamon
½ teaspoon nutmeg
Powdered sugar, optional
cinnamon-sugar, optional
regular or sugar-free maple syrup, optional

Cut a horizontal slot into each piece of bread but do not cut all the way through. Combine the cream cheese and orange extract in a small bowl; mix until completely blended. Spoon about 1 to 1½ teaspoons of cream cheese into each slice of bread and spread evenly. Combine the egg substitute, egg whites, half-and-half, cinnamon, and nutmeg in a medium bowl; blend with an electric mixer until frothy. Spray a large nonstick skillet with cooking spray and heat over medium heat. Carefully soak the bread slices in the egg mixture for 30 seconds; cook 3 to 4 slices at a time, until browned on both sides. Remove from the skillet, wrap in foil and keep warm. Remove the skillet from the heat, spray again with cooking spray, and repeat the process with the remaining bread. Serve French Toast Pockets with powdered sugar, cinnamon-sugar mixture, or syrup, as desired.

Nutrition per serving: Calories 253 · Fat 2.7g · Carbohydrates 39g · Protein 16g · Cholesterol 0mg · Dietary fiber 2g · Sodium 676mg
Exchanges: 3 other carb · ½ fat
Carb Choices: 3

The secret to heart-healthy cooking... there is no secret! Heart-healthy cooking simply means preparing dishes lower in saturated fat, cholesterol, and total fat, as well as reducing sodium.

Fruit and Fiber Breakfast

EASY   *Serves: 4*

3 cups skim milk

2½ teaspoons ground cinnamon, divided

¼ teaspoon nutmeg

2 cups quick-cooking oatmeal

1¼ cups frozen mango chunks, thawed and drained

¼ cup toasted wheat germ

2 tablespoons brown sugar

Combine the milk, cinnamon, and nutmeg in a medium saucepan; bring to a boil, stirring frequently, over medium-high heat. Add the oatmeal; return to a boil. Reduce heat to medium and cook 1 minute, stirring frequently. Add the mango chunks; cook, stirring constantly, until the fruit is heated through and most of the liquid is absorbed. Combine the wheat germ and brown sugar in a small bowl; mix with your fingertips until blended. Sprinkle the mixture over the cooked oatmeal and serve.

Nutrition per serving: Calories 318 • Fat 3.8g • Carbohydrates 59g • Protein 15g • Cholesterol 3mg • Dietary fiber 5g • Sodium 101mg

Exchanges: 1 starch • 1 milk • 1 fruit • 1 other carb

Carb Choices: 4

> Oatmeal contains more soluble fiber than any other food, making it one of the best cholesterol busters you can add to your diet. Studies have shown that barley is just as effective in reducing cholesterol levels and lowering heart attack risk.

Fruit 'n' Yogurt with Kashi

EASY • DO AHEAD   *Serves: 2*

2 cups nonfat vanilla yogurt
2 bananas, cut into ½-inch slices
3 cups seedless grapes, cut in half
1½ cups Kashi Good Friends cereal

Combine yogurt, bananas, and grapes in a bowl and toss until coated. Cover and chill until ready to serve. Divide yogurt/fruit mixture between two bowls; top each with ¾ cup Kashi cereal. Toss lightly and serve.

Nutrition per serving: Calories 335 • Fat 1.4g • Carbohydrates 74g • Protein 12g • Cholesterol 5mg • Dietary fiber 6g • Sodium 144mg

Exchanges: 1 milk • 3 fruit • 1 starch

Carb Choices: 5

Researchers at Tulane University discovered eating one banana a day can boost potassium intake and lower the risk of stroke by 28 percent. Other great potassium sources: one cup of cantaloupe or a baked potato.

Garden Frittata

EASY   *Serves: 4*

1 tablespoon nonfat vegetable
  broth
1½ cups precooked diced
  potatoes
1 cup frozen chopped spinach,
  thawed and drained well
¼ tablespoon chopped green
  onions

¼ cup pimientos, drained and
  dried
1 teaspoon celery seed
1½ cups Vegetable Garden Egg
  Beaters
1 tablespoon nonfat cottage
  cheese

Spray a large nonstick skillet with cooking spray; add the vegetable broth and heat over medium-high heat. Add the potatoes; cook, stirring frequently, for about 5 minutes, until lightly browned. Add the thawed spinach, green onions, and pimientos; cook for 3 to 4 minutes, until the vegetables are softened. Add the celery seed and mix well. Combine the egg substitute and cottage cheese in a medium bowl; mix until blended. Pour the egg mixture into the skillet; cook, lifting the edges of the egg mixture so the uncooked portion can flow underneath. Continue cooking until the eggs are completely set. Cover the skillet and cook for 1 to 2 minutes. Serve immediately.

Nutrition per serving: Calories 120 • Fat 0.3g • Carbohydrates 18g • Protein 12g •
  Cholesterol 0mg • Dietary fiber 3g • Sodium 335mg
Exchanges: ½ starch • 2 vegetable • 1 very lean meat
Carb Choices: 1

> For each 10 grams of fiber you add to your daily diet, you are lowering your risk of coronary disease by 14 percent and decreasing your chances of dying of heart disease by 27 percent.

Huevos Mexicano

EASY   *Serves: 4*

1 cup Southwest-style hash
  brown potatoes
Pepper to taste
¾ cup Southwest Egg Beaters
6 large egg whites
3 tablespoons diced green chiles,
  drained

¼ cup chunky-style salsa
2 tablespoons nonfat half-
  and-half
1 cup nonfat shredded cheddar
  cheese

Preheat the oven to 350 degrees. Lightly spray an 8-inch baking dish with cooking spray. Spread the hash brown potatoes in the bottom of the dish; sprinkle with pepper to taste. Combine the remaining ingredients in a medium bowl and mix until blended and frothy. Pour the mixture over the potatoes; bake for 40 to 45 minutes, until the center is cooked through.

Nutrition per serving: Calories 130 • Fat 0g • Carbohydrates 11g • Protein 19g •
  Cholesterol 0mg • Dietary fiber 1g • Sodium 718mg
Exchanges: 2 very lean meat • ½ starch • 1 vegetable
Carb Choices: 1

Skipping breakfast could be considered a significant health risk. Ramifications of missing the morning meal include: headache and fatigue; increased cholesterol levels; impaired thinking; nutritional deficiency, and greater risk for obesity. Skipping breakfast slows the rate at which your body burns calories, increases high-fat snacking, and leads to vitamin and mineral deficiencies.

Mushroom and Broccoli Frittata

AVERAGE

Serves: 4

¾ cups egg substitute

6 large egg whites

½ teaspoon dried Italian
   seasoning

¼ teaspoon garlic powder

¼ teaspoon pepper

1 tablespoon onion powder

2 cups frozen chopped broccoli,
   thawed and drained

1½ cups sliced mushrooms

1 cup nonfat shredded cheddar
   cheese

Combine the egg substitute, egg whites, Italian seasoning, garlic powder, pepper, and onion powder in a medium bowl; blend until frothy. Wrap a large nonstick skillet handle with heavy-duty foil. Spray the skillet with cooking spray and heat over medium-high heat. Add the broccoli and mushrooms to the skillet; cook, stirring frequently, for 5 to 6 minutes, until softened. Pour the egg mixture over the broccoli and mushrooms; cover and cook over medium heat until the eggs are set, lifting several times so the uncooked eggs run underneath. Preheat the broiler. Place the eggs under the broiler for 1 minute; top with the cheese and broil for 1 to 2 minutes, until the cheese is melted and lightly browned.

Nutrition per serving: Calories 132 · Fat 0.2g · Carbohydrates 11g · Protein 21g ·
   Cholesterol 0mg · Dietary fiber 4g · Sodium 522mg

Exchanges: 2½ very lean meat · 2 vegetable

Carb Choices: 1

Egg whites are always a heart-healthy choice; with 3 grams of protein per white and zero cholesterol, they are a low-calorie, fat-free source of protein.

Pineapple-Orange Muffins

EASY • DO AHEAD • FREEZE   *Serves: 12*

¾ cup crushed pineapple in
  juice, undrained
1 cup nonfat vanilla yogurt
¼ cup egg substitute
2 tablespoons orange juice
¼ cup sugar

½ teaspoon vanilla
1 cup all-purpose flour
1½ cups quick-cooking oatmeal,
  uncooked
1 teaspoon baking powder
½ teaspoon baking soda

Preheat the oven to 350 degrees. Spray muffin tin with cooking spray. Combine the pineapple, yogurt, egg substitute, orange juice, sugar, and vanilla in a large bowl; mix until the ingredients are blended smooth. Combine the flour, oatmeal, baking powder, and baking soda in a zip-top bag; shake to mix well. Add the dry ingredients all at once and mix just until the ingredients are blended and moistened. Fill the muffin cups with batter and bake for 20 to 25 minutes, until a toothpick inserted in the center comes out clean.

Nutrition per serving: Calories 113 • Fat 0.7g • Carbohydrates 23g • Protein 4g • Cholesterol <1mg • Dietary fiber 1g • Sodium 89mg

Exchanges: 2 other carb

Carb Choices: 2

> Eat pineapple for achy joints—pineapple contains bromelain, an enzyme that inhibits the release of chemicals that trigger inflammation.

Pumpkin-Raisin Muffins

EASY • DO AHEAD • FREEZE   *Serves: 12*

1 cup canned pumpkin
¾ cup nonfat vanilla yogurt
⅓ cup sugar
⅓ cup brown sugar
¼ cup egg substitute
1 teaspoon vanilla extract
1 cup crushed Kashi Good
   Friends cereal

¾ cup whole-wheat flour
½ cup all-purpose flour
2 teaspoons baking powder
1½ teaspoons cinnamon
½ cup raisins

Preheat the oven to 350 degrees. Spray a 12-cup muffin tin with cooking spray. Combine the pumpkin, yogurt, sugar, brown sugar, egg substitute, and vanilla in a large bowl; mix well. Combine the crushed cereal, whole-wheat flour, all-purpose flour, baking powder, and cinnamon in a large zip-top bag; shake until the ingredients are well mixed. Gradually add to the pumpkin mixture, stirring just until the ingredients are moistened and blended. Fold in the raisins. Spoon the batter into muffin cups; bake for 20 to 25 minutes, until a toothpick inserted in the center comes out clean. Cool for 5 minutes before removing from pan.

Nutrition per serving: Calories 135 • Fat 0.3g • Carbohydrates 30g • Protein 5g •
   Cholesterol <1mg • Dietary fiber 2g • Sodium 128mg
Exchanges: 2 other carb
Carb Choices: 2

Nutrition-packed superheroes contain antioxidant properties that boost immunity, fight cancer, heart disease, colds, and flu, as well as slow down the aging process. A few of these super foods include berries (blueberries, blackberries, strawberries); leafy greens (spinach, kale); and dried fruits (dried plums, raisins).

Pumpkin Spice Oatmeal

EASY   *Serves: 6*

1½ cups skim milk
1½ cups water
1½ teaspoons pumpkin pie spice
½ teaspoon cinnamon
2 cups quick-cooking oatmeal

1 cup canned pumpkin
¼ cup plus 2 tablespoons brown
  sugar
½ cup raisins

Combine the milk, water, pumpkin pie spice, and cinnamon in a medium saucepan; bring to a boil over medium-high heat. Stir in the oatmeal; return to a boil. Reduce the heat to medium; cook, stirring frequently, for 1 to 2 minutes, until the liquid is absorbed. Remove from the heat; immediately stir in the pumpkin and brown sugar and mix well. Let stand until the oatmeal reaches desired consistency, about 3 to 5 minutes. Fold in the raisins. Serve with additional cinnamon, if desired.

Nutrition per serving: Calories 230 · Fat 2.1g · Carbohydrates 48g · Protein 7g ·
  Cholesterol 1mg · Dietary fiber 3g · Sodium 40mg
Exchanges: 1 other carb · 1 fruit · 1 starch
Carb Choices: 3

High-fiber cereal is an excellent breakfast choice—slowly digested, high-fiber cereal keeps you satisfied longer, keeps blood sugar levels stable, relieves constipation, and reduces fat intake. Skipping breakfast can slow your metabolism by five percent—not only that, but you're setting yourself up for an energy drain! Look for cereal with a minimum of 5 grams of fiber per serving.

Turkey-Vegetable Quiche

EASY ▪ DO AHEAD   *Serves: 4*

1-pound 4-ounce package sliced
  home fries
1 cup nonfat shredded cheddar
  cheese
1 cup nonfat cottage cheese
½ cup egg substitute
4 large egg whites

¾ cup diced cooked turkey or
  chicken
¼ cup sliced green onions
⅓ pound fresh asparagus, cut
  into 1-inch pieces
2 tablespoons flour
Pepper to taste

Preheat the oven to 375 degrees. Spray a 9x13-inch baking dish with cooking spray. Line the bottom of the baking dish with potato slices. Combine the remaining ingredients in a large bowl; mix until blended. Pour the egg mixture over the potatoes and bake, uncovered for 55 to 60 minutes, until a toothpick inserted in the center comes out clean. Remove from the oven and let the quiche sit for 5 minutes before slicing into squares.

Nutrition per serving: Calories 273 • Fat 0.8g • Carbohydrates 37g • Protein 27g •
  Cholesterol 18mg • Dietary fiber 2g • Sodium 793mg
Exchanges: 2 starch • 3 very lean meat • 1 vegetable
Carb Choices: 2

To trim asparagus, bend the stalk; it will break off at the spot where it becomes too tough to eat.

Salads and Soups

Salads

Salads can provide the same satiating sensations as soup, as long as you make healthy food choices. A salad can make or break a week's worth of weight watching if you aren't equipped with salad smarts! Deciphering the colorful language of salads can save your "butt" from unwanted calories and fat. Turn a side-dish salad into a main meal by adding lean meat, fish, or poultry.

The good news . . . a salad is (potentially)

- low in calories
- low in fat
- bursting with vital nutrients
- full of fat fighters

- a plateful of fiber, vitamins, and minerals
- a great way to meet your daily vegetable quota
- a healthy choice

The bad news . . . a salad is frequently misunderstood, miscalculated, and the ultimate diet disaster on a plate!

Color counts! Naturally low in calories and fat, you get a lot more for your money from the greenest greens.

TYPE OF GREENS (NUTRITION PER 1 CUP)	CALCIUM (MG)	POTASSIUM (MG)	VITAMIN C (MG)	VITAMIN A (MG)
Romaine	20	162	13.40	146
Cabbage	32	172	33	8
Dandelion greens	103	218	19.30	770
Endive	26	158	3.20	102
Spinach	56	312	16	376
Kale	90	299	80.40	596
Radicchio	8	120	3.20	2
Watercress	40	112	14.60	160
Swiss chard	18	136	10.80	118
Arugula	32	74	0	48

Filling you up without filling you out! Simply stuffing your salad plate with "pile ons" rather than "take offs" can save you over 700 calories and more than 60 grams of fat! Most of these foods are high in water content and fiber so you leave the table feeling full and satisfied without overloading on unwanted calories and fat.

Pile on These Ingredients for Maximum Satiety and Health Benefits!	Take These Ingredients off for Optimal Savings!	What You'll Be Saving ...
Cruciferous vegetables with cancer-fighting nitrogen compounds, vitamin C, and folate Examples: Brussels sprouts, broccoli, cabbage, cauliflower, collard greens, kale, kohlrabi, mustard, rutabaga, turnips	2 tablespoons regular croutons	140 calories 6 grams of fat
Canned beans for soluble fiber Examples: garbanzo beans, kidney beans, pinto beans, navy beans	2 tablespoons chow mein noodles	30 calories 2 grams fat
Dried fruits for potassium, vitamin A, and beta-carotene Examples: chopped dried figs, dates, apricots, raisins	¼ avocado	84 calories 8 grams fat
Fresh fruits for fiber, potassium, and vitamin C Examples: apples, nectarines, peaches, grapes, berries, kiwifruit, mango, papaya, pineapple	2 tablespoons coconut	35 calories 3 grams fat
Frozen vegetables for calcium, potassium, and vitamin C Examples: peas, corn	2 tablespoons granola	74 calories 4 grams fat
Tomatoes for potassium, vitamin A and C	5 olives	26 calories 2 grams fat
Cooked grains for protein, potassium, and iron Examples: quinoa, rice, couscous, barley	2 tablespoons sunflower seeds	104 calories 10 grams fat

Pile on These Ingredients for Maximum Satiety and Health Benefits!	Take These Ingredients off for Optimal Savings!	What You'll Be Saving . . .
Fresh vegetables for fiber, beta-carotene, potassium, and vitamin C Examples: carrots, jicama, cucumbers, bell peppers, red onions	2 tablespoons cheddar cheese	57 calories 5 grams fat
Fresh herbs Examples: basil, chervil, chives, dill, marjoram, oregano, parsley, tarragon, thyme	2 tablespoons bacon bits	54 calories 3 grams fat

Are you drowning (your greens) in dressing? The average woman between the ages of nineteen and fifty packs on more fat grams from salad dressing than from any other food in her diet! Stick with fat-free dressings, flavored vinegars, lemon juice, or fat-free yogurt spiked with herbs. This one simple change can help you cut up to 27 grams of fat per 2 tablespoon serving.

The Satiety Scoop on Salads

Researchers from Pennsylvania State University found that starting lunch with a low-fat salad (less than 14 percent calories from fat) can reduce the total number of calories consumed in the meal. Consuming 3 cups of low-fat salad resulted in a 12 percent overall reduction in lunch calories compared with 7 percent fewer calories for those who ate only 1½ cups of salad. The most surprising news was that participants felt fuller on three cups of salad weighing in at 100 calories than the same portion with 400 calories and more fat.

ALL YOU EVER WANTED TO KNOW ABOUT CHICKEN BUT WERE AFRAID TO ASK . . .

- One of the most versatile food items, chicken can be baked, broiled, grilled, sautéed, stir-fried, boiled, microwaved, or poached. Boneless, skinless chicken breasts or tenderloins prepared without oil or butter are an excellent source of protein and provide a significant amount of B vitamins, iron, potassium, and zinc.
- A 3-ounce serving of chicken provides almost half of your daily protein requirement.
- Surprise, surprise! A research study at the University of Minnesota found that no significant fat is transferred from the skin to the meat when chicken is cooked. So go ahead and leave the skin on while cooking, but take it off before your first bite.
- Safety counts! Always cook chicken until the juices run clear when pierced with a fork.

Caesar Crab Salad

EASY • DO AHEAD *Serves: 4*

8 ounces bow-tie pasta
15-ounce can cannellini (white
  kidney beans), drained
1 cup grape tomatoes
2 6-ounce cans crabmeat,
  drained well

½ cup nonfat Caesar salad
  dressing
1 tablespoon nonfat Parmesan
  cheese

Cook the pasta according to package directions; drain and cool. Combine the cooked pasta, beans, tomatoes, and crabmeat in a medium bowl; toss lightly to mix. Pour the dressing over the top and toss until the ingredients are coated. Sprinkle with Parmesan cheese just before serving.

Nutrition per serving: Calories 423 • Fat 1.4g • Carbohydrates 71g • Protein 31g •
  Cholesterol 105mg • Dietary fiber 6g • Sodium 1,149mg
Exchanges: 4 starch • 2 vegetable • 2 very lean meat
Carb Choices: 5

You need more than forty different nutrients for good health, and no single food supplies them all. Include whole-grain bread, as well as fruits, vegetables, meat, and dairy products in your daily meals.

Chef's Ranch Salad

EASY • DO AHEAD   *Serves: 4*

6 cups baby spinach leaves

6 cups chopped romaine lettuce

1½ cup diced cauliflower florets

1 cup sliced bell peppers

1 cup sliced mushrooms

1 cup shredded carrots

1 cup grape tomatoes

4 hard-cooked egg whites, chopped

12-ounce package cooked chicken breast cuts

4 ounces whole nonfat mozzarella cheese, cut into thin strips

½ cup nonfat croutons

½ cup nonfat ranch salad dressing

Combine all the ingredients except the salad dressing in a large bowl; toss to mix. Pour the dressing over the top and toss until the ingredients are coated. If preparing ahead, add the croutons with the salad dressing.

Nutrition per serving: Calories 314 • Fat 4.4g • Carbohydrates 25g • Protein 42g • Cholesterol 64mg • Dietary fiber 6g • Sodium 790mg

Exchanges: 3 vegetable • 2 lean meat • 2 very lean meat • ½ other carb

Carb Choices: 2

Adding just one extra serving (a medium-sized piece or 4 ounces) of fruits or vegetables to your daily diet can reduce your risk of heart disease by 4 percent.

Chicken and Rice Salad

EASY • DO AHEAD   *Serves: 4*

1 cup nonfat mayonnaise
2 tablespoons diced red bell
   pepper
¾ cup diced celery
¾ cup diced jicama
12-ounce package cooked
   chicken breast cuts

1½ cups frozen peas, thawed and
   drained
1½ cups cooked rice
¼ teaspoon pepper
16-ounce package mixed salad
   greens

Combine the mayonnaise, bell pepper, celery, jicama, chicken, peas, rice, and pepper in a medium bowl; toss carefully, cover, and refrigerate at least 1 hour. Serve the chicken and rice salad over mixed salad greens.

Nutrition per serving: Calories 347 • Fat 4.3g • Carbohydrates 46g • Protein 30g • Cholesterol 64mg • Dietary fiber 5g • Sodium 549mg
Exchanges: 2 starch • 2 vegetable • 2 lean meat • 1 very lean meat
Carb Choices: 3

You can refrigerate cooked rice in a tightly sealed container for up to one week or freeze for up to six months.

Chicken-Vegetable Pasta Salad

EASY • DO AHEAD   *Serves: 4*

½ cup nonfat mayonnaise
1⅔ cups nonfat chicken broth
¼ cup nonfat Parmesan cheese
1 teaspoon celery seed
12-ounce package cooked
   chicken breast cuts

3 cups whole-wheat macaroni,
   cooked and drained (keep hot)
½ cup sliced mushrooms
¾ cup chopped red onion
1 cup grape tomatoes, cut in half

Combine the mayonnaise, chicken broth, Parmesan cheese, and celery seed in a medium bowl; mix well and set aside. Combine the chicken, hot cooked macaroni, mushrooms, red onions, and tomatoes in a large bowl; toss lightly to mix. Pour the dressing over the top and mix well. Cover and refrigerate at least 4 hours, or overnight. Stir lightly before serving.

Nutrition per serving: Calories 462 • Fat 4.5g • Carbohydrates 71g • Protein 38g • Cholesterol 60mg • Dietary fiber 1g • Sodium 1,469mg

Exchanges: 1 other carb • 3 starch • 2 vegetable • 2 lean meat • 1 very lean meat

Carb Choices: 5

Don't store tomatoes in the refrigerator—tomatoes hate the cold because the enzyme that gives them their flavor is destroyed below 50 degrees. You can keep tomatoes for up to seven days right on your kitchen counter.

Honey-Dijon Pasta Salad with Tuna

EASY • DO AHEAD   *Serves: 4*

8 ounces small shell whole-wheat
    pasta
12 ounces canned tuna in water,
    drained well
¾ cup diced bell pepper (any
    variety)
½ cup diced celery

¼ cup canned water chestnuts,
    drained and finely diced
½ cup chopped red onion
¾ cup nonfat honey-Dijon salad
    dressing (or other nonfat
    dressing of choice)

Cook and drain the pasta according to package directions. Combine the pasta, tuna, bell pepper, celery, water chestnuts, and red onion in a medium bowl. Pour the dressing over the salad and toss to coat. Cover and refrigerate until ready to serve.

Nutrition per serving: Calories 383 • Fat 2.9g • Carbohydrates 58g • Protein 32g •
    Cholesterol 36mg • Dietary fiber 1g • Sodium 757mg
Exchanges: 3 very lean meat • 2 starch • 3 vegetable • 1 other starch
Carb Choices: 4

Take the guesswork out of vegetable math: 1 medium onion (5 ounces) = ½ cup chopped; 1 medium bell pepper (3 ounces) = ¾ cup chopped or 1 cup strips; and 1 medium tomato (5 ounces) = ½ cup seeded and chopped.

Honey Yogurt Fruit Bowl

EASY • DO AHEAD   *Serves: 4*

2 bananas, cut into 1-inch slices

1 cup fresh pineapple chunks,
    drained well

2 oranges, peeled, seeded, and
    sliced thin

1 cup seedless grapes (red or
    green)

¾ cup nonfat vanilla yogurt

1 tablespoon honey

1 tablespoon sliced almonds,
    optional

Combine the bananas, pineapple, oranges, and grapes in a medium bowl. Combine the vanilla yogurt and honey in a small bowl; mix well. Pour the yogurt mixture over the top and toss until coated. Cover and refrigerate 30 minutes before serving. Sprinkle with almonds just before serving, if desired.

Nutrition per serving: Calories 162 • Fat 1.6g • Carbohydrates 37g • Protein 3g •
    Cholesterol 1mg • Dietary fiber 4g • Sodium 28mg

Exchanges: 2 fruit • ½ other carb

Carb Choices: 2

British researchers found that snacking on an orange a day cuts your risk of dying from heart disease by 20 percent, regardless of age, blood pressure, or cholesterol levels. The study showed that adding just 50 grams of vitamin C to your daily diet (one orange, 3 ounces orange juice, or 3 ounces sliced green pepper) is enough to keep your heart healthy for life.

Nutty Fruit Salad

EASY • DO AHEAD   *Serves: 4*

1½ cups nonfat vanilla yogurt	1 banana, peeled and sliced thin
1 tablespoon honey	½ pound fresh pineapple, cut in
3 cups diced apple	chunks and drained well
¼ pound seedless grapes	2 tablespoons chopped walnuts

Combine the yogurt and honey in a small bowl; mix well. Combine the remaining ingredients in a large bowl; pour the yogurt mixture over the top and toss to mix. Cover and refrigerate 15 to 20 minutes before serving.

Nutrition per serving: Calories 180 • Fat 2.9g • Carbohydrates 37g • Protein 5g •
Cholesterol 2mg • Dietary fiber 3g • Sodium 54mg
Exchanges: ½ fat • 2 fruit • ½ other carb
Carb Choices: 2

> Studies show that people who eat nuts regularly have less heart disease and other illnesses than people who don't. The heart-healthy monounsaturated fats they contain are also better for your joints than polyunsaturated fats. The key is moderation: Nuts are high in calories and fat!

Pita Stuffed with Spinach Salad

EASY • DO AHEAD   *Serves: 4*

6 cups baby spinach
½ cup sliced mushrooms
¼ cup diced red onion
⅔ cups garbanzo beans, drained
1 tablespoon packaged bacon
  crumbles
1 medium orange, peeled, seeded,
  and chopped

1 tablespoon nonfat or reduced-
  fat crumbled feta cheese
½ cup nonfat ranch salad
  dressing
4 whole-wheat pita pockets, cut
  in half

Combine the spinach, mushrooms, onion, garbanzo beans, bacon crumbles, orange, and cheese in a large bowl; toss to mix. Pour the dressing over the top and toss until the ingredients are coated. Stuff the spinach salad into the pita pockets and serve. Salad (without dressing) can be prepared ahead of time, covered, and refrigerated until ready to serve.

Nutrition per serving: Calories 236 • Fat 1.7g • Carbohydrates 45g • Protein 10g •
  Cholesterol 0mg • Dietary fiber 4g • Sodium 788mg
Exchanges: 1 other carb • 1 starch • 3 vegetable
Carb Choices: 3

Australian researchers found that subjects who ate fiber-rich breads such as whole-wheat buns felt satisfied sooner—and ate less in a subsequent two-hour period—than those who ate refined white bread.

Poppy Seed Coleslaw

EASY • DO AHEAD   *Serves: 6*

½ cup nonfat mayonnaise
3 tablespoons apple cider
1 tablespoon honey
¾ teaspoon celery seed
⅛ teaspoon salt

1 tablespoon poppy seeds
Pepper to taste
6 cups shredded cabbage mix
1 cup shredded carrots

Combine the mayonnaise, apple cider, honey, celery seed, salt, poppy seeds, and pepper in a medium bowl; mix until creamy and smooth. Combine the cabbage mix and carrots in a large bowl; toss to mix. Pour the dressing over the top and toss until the ingredients are coated. Cover and refrigerate 3 to 4 hours before serving.

Nutrition per serving: Calories 66 • Fat 0.8g • Carbohydrates 14g • Protein 2g •
  Cholesterol 0mg • Dietary fiber 2g • Sodium 208mg
Exchanges: 1 vegetable • ½ other carb
Carb Choices: 1

Red cabbage contains anthocyanins, anti-inflammatory antioxidants that help prevent heart disease.

Spicy Romaine Shrimp Salad

EASY   *Serves: 4*

6 cups romaine lettuce
6 ounces frozen pea pods,
  thawed and drained
15-ounce can baby corn, drained
8 ounces cooked medium shrimp
1 cup bell pepper strips
½ cup diced water chestnuts,
  drained well

½ cup nonfat French or Catalina
  salad dressing
1 tablespoon low-sodium soy
  sauce
⅛ teaspoon cayenne

Combine the lettuce, pea pods, corn, shrimp, pepper strips, and water chestnuts in a medium bowl; toss lightly. Combine the remaining ingredients and mix well. Pour the dressing over the salad; toss lightly and serve.

Nutrition per serving: Calories 174 • Fat 2.8g • Carbohydrates 23g • Protein 14g • Cholesterol 87mg • Dietary fiber 3g • Sodium 520mg

Exchanges: 2 vegetable • 1½ lean meat • ½ other carb

Carb Choices: 2

> Sugar snap peas are one of the richest vegetable sources of thiamin (vitamin B_1), which speeds the body's conversion of carbohydrates into energy.

Superstar Bean Salad

EASY • DO AHEAD   *Serves: 4*

½ cup canned black beans,   ½ cup diced red onion
  rinsed and drained   6 tablespoons apricot preserves
½ cup canned Great Northern   2 tablespoons cider vinegar
  beans, rinsed and drained   ¾ teaspoon Splenda or sugar
1 cup canned red kidney beans,
  rinsed and drained

Combine the beans and onions in a medium bowl and toss to mix. Combine the preserves, vinegar, and Splenda in a small bowl; mix until smooth. Spoon the mixture over the beans and toss until coated. Cover and refrigerate at least 8 hours or overnight.

Nutrition per serving: Calories 215 • Fat 0.4g • Carbohydrates 46g • Protein 8g •
   Cholesterol 0mg • Dietary fiber 5g • Sodium 329mg
Exchanges: 2 starch • 1 other carb
Carb Choices: 3

Researchers from Tulane University and the National Heart, Lung, and Blood Institute found that people who ate legumes at least four times a week were 22 percent less likely to develop heart disease than those who ate them less than once a week.

Tarragon Potato Salad

EASY • DO AHEAD   *Serves: 8*

¼ cup nonfat plain yogurt
¼ cup nonfat sour cream
¼ cup nonfat mayonnaise
1½ tablespoons nonfat ranch
    seasoning and dressing mix
1½ pounds small red potatoes
¼ teaspoon dried tarragon
3 tablespoons apple cider
    vinegar

1 cup diced cucumber
½ cup diced jicama
½ cup diced bell pepper
2 teaspoons dried parsley
2 teaspoons dried dill
2 teaspoons dried chives

Combine the yogurt, sour cream, mayonnaise, and seasoning mix in a food processor or blender; mix until smooth. Pour into a bowl, cover, and refrigerate several hours or overnight. Place the potatoes in a large saucepan; cover with water. Bring to a boil over high heat; reduce heat to low, cover, and simmer 20 to 25 minutes, until potatoes are tender. Drain the potatoes and cool for 10 to 15 minutes. Slice the potatoes and place in a medium bowl; sprinkle with tarragon and drizzle with cider vinegar. Toss the potatoes and let stand until completely cooled. Add the remaining ingredients to the potatoes. Toss gently with refrigerated dressing. Cover and refrigerate at least 1 hour before serving.

Nutrition per serving: Calories 98 • Fat 0.1g • Carbohydrates 23g • Protein 3g •
    Cholesterol <1mg • Dietary fiber 1g • Sodium 94mg
Exchanges: ½ starch • 1 vegetable • ½ other carb
Carb Choices: 2

> Remove cucumber seeds easily: Cut cucumber lengthwise in half and scrape a teaspoon or melon baller down the middle of each half.

Tarragon Shrimp Salad

EASY • DO AHEAD   *Serves: 4*

½ pound asparagus
1 pound medium cooked shrimp,
    peeled
¾ cup diced red bell pepper
¼ cup diced celery
⅓ cup chopped green onions

½ cup nonfat mayonnaise
2 tablespoons lemon juice
1 teaspoon dried tarragon
2 teaspoons grated lemon peel
⅛ teaspoon cayenne
6 cups shredded lettuce, optional

Clean the asparagus, break off ends, and cut into 1-inch pieces. Wrap the asparagus pieces in paper towels; microwave on high heat for 3 minutes, until tender crisp. Combine the asparagus, cooked shrimp, bell pepper, celery, and onions in a large bowl. Combine the remaining ingredients in a medium bowl and mix until completely blended. Spoon the mayonnaise mixture over the shrimp and toss until the ingredients are evenly coated. Cover and refrigerate for 30 to 45 minutes; serve on shredded lettuce, if desired.

Nutrition per serving: Calories 133 • Fat 1.2g • Carbohydrates 9g • Protein 21g •
    Cholesterol 174mg • Dietary fiber 1g • Sodium 419mg
Exchanges: 2½ very lean meat • 2 vegetable
Carb Choices: 1

Some of the best low-calorie, low-fat fish choices include: cod (119 calories/ 0.9 grams fat); skate (131 calories/0.9 grams fat); yellowfin tuna (123 calories/ 1 gram fat); shrimp (112 calories/1.2 grams fat); sole and flounder (133 calories/1.7 grams fat).

Wonderful Waldorf Salad

EASY • DO AHEAD   *Serves: 4*

2 pears, cored and diced
1 Granny Smith apple, cored
  and diced
¼ cup lemon juice, divided
½ cup water
¾ cup diced celery

1 kiwifruit, peeled and diced
2 tablespoons toasted walnuts,
  chopped fine
⅔ cup nonfat vanilla yogurt
2 tablespoons nonfat mayonnaise
2 teaspoons sugar

Place the diced pears and apples in a large bowl; combine 2 tablespoons of lemon juice and water and drizzle over the fruit. Cover and refrigerate for 10 to 15 minutes. Drain the fruit and return to the bowl; add the celery, kiwifruit, and walnuts and toss to mix. Combine the yogurt, the remaining 2 tablespoons of lemon juice, mayonnaise, and sugar in a small bowl; mix until smooth and blended. Pour the dressing over the fruit mixture; toss to coat. Cover and refrigerate for 1 to 3 hours before serving.

Nutrition per serving: Calories 139 • Fat 2.7g • Carbohydrates 29g • Protein 3g •
Cholesterol 1mg • Dietary fiber 4g • Sodium 97mg
Exchanges: ½ fat • 1½ fruit • ½ other carb
Carb Choices: 2

> A study at the University of California at Davis found that consuming three walnuts a day, rich in polyunsaturated fat, reduced "bad" LDL cholesterol levels by 27 percent.

Tortilla Roll-up with Black Beans

EASY ▪ DO AHEAD   *Serves: 6*

15-ounce can black beans, rinsed
  and drained
3 tablespoons lemon juice
1½ teaspoons chili powder
½ cup finely chopped jicama
¼ cup diced red onion
½ cup chopped bell pepper, red
  or green
¼ cup diced green chiles

¾ cup nonfat shredded cheddar
  cheese
6 low-fat whole-wheat flour
  tortillas
Chopped tomato
Shredded lettuce, optional
Chopped cilantro, optional
Nonfat sour cream, optional
Salsa, optional

Place the beans in a medium bowl; mash until smooth. Add the lemon juice
and chili powder; mix well. Stir in the jicama, onion, bell pepper, and green
chiles. Cover and refrigerate at least 1 hour. When ready to serve: Spread each
tortilla with the bean mixture; top with garnishes as desired.

Nutrition per serving: Calories 221 • Fat 0.8g • Carbohydrates 41g • Protein 13g •
  Cholesterol 0mg • Dietary fiber 5g • Sodium 827mg
Exchanges: 2 starch • 2 vegetable • ½ very lean meat
Carb Choices: 3

> Keep tortillas from cracking when making wraps by rolling them loosely. If
> they do crack, warm the tortillas in a microwave oven according to package
> directions.

Soups

Soup can be a magical meal—it fills you up with a lighter feel! Recent research shows that adding water to the food you eat helps reduce calorie intake. Broth-based soups are one of the best ways to fill up without filling out. In a research study, women who ate a bowl of chicken soup felt fuller than those who ate chicken casserole plus a glass of water, even though both meals contained exactly the same ingredients and quantities. The soup-eaters tended to be less hungry and ate fewer calories at their next meal than those who ate the casserole and drank water separately. Women consumed almost 400 fewer calories a day when they started their meal with soup. Working on the energy density concept, especially when based on low-calorie, low-saturated fat ingredients, soups are versatile choices with a high "fill factor." Whether you start with a can, bouillon cubes, or make your own broth, you can build a healthy one-dish meal by adding a variety of beans, vegetables, and lean meats. Quick to prepare, easy to make-ahead and reheat, soups are one of the most easy and nutritious dishes, made with ingredients available in any healthy kitchen.

Soups are Satisfying!

- Soups span the international globe, satisfying taste buds everywhere! From patsas and fasolada in Greece to Italian minestrone, French bouillabiasse and onion soup, Russian borscht and Spanish gazpacho, soups are satisfying!
- Begin with a broth base and let your imagination run wild with a slew of lean meats, beans, vegetables, fruits, and whole grains.
- Blend ingredients for a smooth creamy texture; thicken with starchy vegetables (potatoes, carrots, flour, or cornstarch); convert into a full meal with whole grains and beans; and garnish with an array of ingredients from low-fat cheese and croutons to freshly chopped spices.

- Most soups can be stored in the refrigerator for three to four days or several weeks in the freezer. Soups with fish or seafood should be consumed within one to two days.
- Hot, cold, or mildly temperate, soups satisfy the flavors of every season.

Chicken and Rice Tortilla Soup

EASY • DO AHEAD • FREEZE   *Serves: 8*

8 cups water
9-ounce package Bear Creek
  Tortilla Soup Mix
2 15-ounce cans diced tomatoes
  with onions and garlic,
  well drained
11-ounce can corn kernels,
  drained
1 cup frozen seasoning
  vegetables (onion, celery, bell
  pepper)

1 cup cooked brown rice
1 pound boneless, skinless
  chicken breasts, cooked
  and cubed
1 cup nonfat shredded cheddar
  cheese
Chopped red onions, optional
Baked tortilla strips, optional
Nonfat sour cream, optional
Green onions, optional

Pour the water into a large saucepan or Dutch oven and bring to a boil over high heat. Add the tortilla soup mix as directed on the package, breaking up the pieces. Add the diced tomatoes, corn, seasoning vegetables, cooked rice, and cubed chicken; bring to a boil over high heat. Reduce heat to low, cover, and simmer for 10 to 20 minutes, stirring occasionally. Ladle soup into bowls; top with 2 tablespoons of cheese and the optional ingredients as desired.

Nutrition per serving: Calories 294 • Fat 3.8g • Carbohydrates 41g • Protein 26g • Cholesterol 43mg • Dietary fiber 6g • Sodium 1,211
Exchanges: 2 vegetable • 2 starch • 2 very lean meat • ½ fat
Carb Choices: 3

> Removing the skin from poultry, trimming fat from meat, and consuming fewer chips can cut as many as 560 calories and 15 grams of saturated fat from your daily intake.

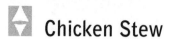 # Chicken Stew

EASY • DO AHEAD • FREEZE   *Serves: 8*

2 pounds boneless, skinless
   chicken breasts
½ cup nonfat chicken broth
½ cup water
1 teaspoon minced garlic
1 tablespoon minced onion
   flakes
½ teaspoon pepper
2 15½-ounce cans diced
   tomatoes, drained

½ teaspoon basil
½ teaspoon Mrs. Dash seasoning
¼ cup diced celery
1-pound 4-ounce package
   precooked potato cubes
10-ounce package frozen baby
   carrots, thawed and drained
2 bay leaves

Combine the chicken breasts, chicken broth, water, garlic, onion flakes, pepper, tomatoes, basil, and Mrs. Dash seasoning in a large nonstick skillet. Bring to a boil over medium-high heat; reduce heat to low, cover, and simmer for 25 to 30 minutes. Add the diced celery, potato cubes, carrots, and bay leaves; cook over medium heat for 10 minutes. Reduce heat to low, cover, and simmer for 15 minutes, until the chicken and vegetables are cooked through. Remove the bay leaf and serve.

Nutrition per serving: Calories 274 • Fat 0.5g • Carbohydrates 22g • Protein 34g •
   Cholesterol 85mg • Dietary fiber 3g • Sodium 306mg
Exchanges: 4 very lean meat • 1 starch • 2 vegetable
Carb Choices: 1

The three most critical moves to protect your heart include: Stop smoking, exercise regularly, and watch the fat. Following a heart-healthy diet is more about what you *do* eat than what you *don't*.

Curried Lentil Soup

EASY · DO AHEAD   *Serves: 4*

1 cup dried lentils, rinsed and drained	¼ cup tomato sauce
2 cups water	2 tablespoons sugar
2 cups nonfat vegetable broth	1½ teaspoons vinegar
2¼ cups shredded carrots	½ teaspoon curry powder
1 large celery stalk, thinly sliced	Pepper to taste

Combine the lentils, water, and vegetable broth in a large saucepan; bring to a boil over medium-high heat. Reduce heat to medium low; skim foam from the top. Add the remaining ingredients and mix well. Cook over medium-low heat, stirring occasionally, for 45 to 50 minutes, until the lentils are tender. Season with pepper.

Nutrition per serving: Calories 227 · Fat 0.8g · Carbohydrates 42g · Protein 16g · Cholesterol 0mg · Dietary fiber 3g · Sodium 430mg

Exchanges: 2 starch · 3 vegetable

Carb Choices: 3

> One serving of dried beans a day can reduce cholesterol by up to 10 percent; beans not only contain compounds that may reduce clotting and improve blood-vessel function, but their high-fiber content may reduce the risk of coronary heart disease by 30 percent.

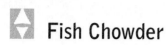 # Fish Chowder

EASY   *Serves: 4*

3 cups plus 2 tablespoons nonfat chicken broth	⅛ teaspoon basil
1 cup sliced celery	Dash of ground red pepper
1 cup diced onion	½ pound cod, cut into ½-inch cubes
1 cup sliced carrots	½ cup evaporated skim milk

Spray a large saucepan with cooking spray; add 2 tablespoons of the broth and heat over medium-high heat. Add the celery and onions; cook, stirring frequently, until the vegetables are softened. Add the remaining 3 cups of broth, carrots, basil, and red pepper. Bring to a boil over high heat; reduce heat to low, cover, and simmer for 15 to 20 minutes, until the vegetables are tender. Add the fish; cook for 5 to 7 minutes. Stir in the evaporated milk; cook, stirring constantly, until blended and heated through.

Nutrition per serving: Calories 122 · Fat 1g · Carbohydrates 12g · Protein 16g · Cholesterol 22mg · Dietary fiber 3g · Sodium 741mg

Exchanges: 2 very lean meat · 2 vegetable

Carb Choices: 1

Onions contain several medicinal compounds, including bioflavonoids, which maximize immunity and fight cancer and heart disease.

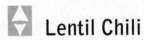

Lentil Chili

EASY • DO AHEAD • FREEZE   *Serves: 6*

2½ cups nonfat vegetable broth

2½ cups boiling water

1 pound dry lentils, rinsed
  and dried

28 ounces diced tomatoes with
  garlic and onion, lightly
  drained

1½ tablespoons chili powder

1 cup chopped onion

½ cup chopped celery

½ teaspoon crushed garlic

Combine the broth and water in a large soup pot; bring to a boil over high heat. Add the lentils, cover, and simmer for 30 to 45 minutes; do not drain. Add the diced tomatoes, chili powder, onion, celery, and garlic. Bring to a boil over medium-high heat; reduce heat to low, cover, and simmer for 30 to 45 minutes, until the lentils are tender. Lentil chili can be served alone or over baked potato, pasta, or rice.

Nutrition per serving: Calories 309 • Fat 1.3g • Carbohydrates 51g • Protein 24g • Cholesterol 0mg • Dietary fiber 3g • Sodium 562mg

Exchanges: 3 starch • 2 vegetable

Carb Choices: 3

Garlic contributes to lowering blood pressure. When garlic is crushed, it produces ajoene, a compound that helps thin blood, reducing the risk of stroke.

Maestro Minestrone

EASY · DO AHEAD   *Serves: 6*

2 cups plus 2 tablespoons nonfat
   chicken broth
2 cups chopped carrots
1 cup chopped onion
1 cup chopped celery
2½ teaspoons crushed garlic
28-ounce can diced tomatoes
   with garlic and onion,
   undrained

1 teaspoon Italian seasoning
2 cups baby spinach
15-ounce can cannellini beans,
   rinsed and drained
⅔ cup cooked orzo

Spray a large saucepan with cooking spray; add 2 tablespoons of the broth and heat over medium-high heat. Add the carrots, onion, celery, and garlic; cook, stirring frequently, over medium-high heat until the vegetables are tender (about 8 to 10 minutes). Add the tomatoes (with juice), remaining broth, and Italian seasoning; bring to a boil over high heat. Reduce heat to low, cover, and simmer for 30 minutes. Add the baby spinach; cover and cook over low heat for 5 to 6 minutes, until the spinach is softened. Add the beans and cooked orzo; heat over medium heat for 3 to 4 minutes, until completely heated through.

Nutrition per serving: Calories 177 · Fat 0.7g · Carbohydrates 33g · Protein 10g · Cholesterol 0mg · Dietary fiber 4g · Sodium 555mg
Exchanges: 4 vegetable · 1 starch
Carb Choices: 2

Tomatoes are the top source of lycopene, an antioxidant that prevents heart disease by reducing "bad" LDL cholesterol and may reduce the harmful effects of ultraviolet rays to prevent sun damage.

Peachy Summer Soup

EASY · DO AHEAD   *Serves: 4*

1½ cups diced cantaloupe	2 teaspoons lime juice
1½ cups diced honeydew melon	1 cup diced peaches
½ cup nonfat peach yogurt	1 cup blueberries
½ cup peach nectar	1 cup sliced strawberries
2 tablespoons sugar	

Combine the cantaloupe, honeydew melon, yogurt, nectar, sugar, and lime juice in a food processor or blender; process until smooth. Pour the soup mixture into a large bowl; add the peaches, blueberries, and strawberries. Mix well; cover and refrigerate for 4 to 6 hours before serving.

Nutrition per serving: Calories 144 · Fat 0.5g · Carbohydrates 36g · Protein 3g · Cholesterol 1mg · Dietary fiber 4g · Sodium 34mg

Exchanges: 2½ fruit

Carb Choices: 2

Eating more healthfully at home involves three main tasks: being prepared with necessary items and wholesome ingredients on hand; preparing foods in the most healthful and tasty way; and keeping fresh, healthy snacks readily available.

Potato-Squash Soup

EASY ▪ DO AHEAD

Serves: 6

2½ cups plus 1 tablespoon
  nonfat chicken or vegetable
  broth
1 cup frozen diced onion
1 Granny Smith apple, peeled
  and diced
1 cup packaged precooked diced
  potatoes

½ teaspoon dried thyme
¼ teaspoon dried basil
⅛ teaspoon ground red pepper
12-ounce package frozen cooked
  squash
½ cup nonfat half-and-half
Pepper to taste

Spray a large saucepan with cooking spray; add 1 tablespoon of broth and heat over medium-high heat. Add the onions; cook, stirring frequently, until the onions are softened. Add the remaining 2½ cups of broth, diced apple, potatoes, thyme, basil, and red pepper. Bring to a boil over high heat; add the frozen squash. Reduce the heat to low, cover, and simmer for 10 to 15 minutes, until the vegetables are softened. Working in several batches, transfer the soup to a food processor or blender and puree until smooth and creamy. Return the soup to the saucepan; add the half-and-half; cook, stirring constantly, over medium heat until the soup is heated through.

Nutrition per serving: Calories 88 • Fat 0.4g • Carbohydrates 19g • Protein 2g • - Cholesterol 0mg • Dietary fiber 2g • Sodium 330mg

Exchanges: 1 starch

Carb Choices: 1

Top apple choices for eating: Red Delicious, McIntosh, Granny Smith, Empire, and Golden Delicious. Top apple choices for pies or applesauce: Jonathon, Newton, and Gravenstein. Top apple choices for baking: Rome Beauty, Northern Spy, Winesap, and York Imperial.

Quick-Cooking Vegetable Bean and Rice Soup

EASY • DO AHEAD   *Serves: 4*

**6 cups nonfat chicken or
   vegetable broth**
**10-ounce package frozen
   carrots, whole, sliced, or diced**
1 zucchini, diced
**16-ounce can Great Northern
   beans, undrained**

1½ cups quick-cooking rice
**¼ teaspoon each: oregano, basil,
   thyme, rosemary**
Dash of cayenne
**4 tablespoons nonfat Parmesan
   cheese**

Bring the broth to a boil in a large saucepan; add the frozen carrots and cook for 3 minutes. Add the zucchini, beans, rice, oregano, basil, thyme, rosemary, and cayenne. Cook over medium-high heat until the zucchini and carrots are tender and the rice is cooked through (about 5 minutes). Divide the soup into four bowls and sprinkle each with 1 tablespoon of Parmesan cheese before serving.

Nutrition per serving: Calories 323 • Fat 1.5g • Carbohydrates 59g • Protein 18g •
   Cholesterol 0mg • Dietary fiber 4g • Sodium 1,269mg
Exchanges: 3 vegetable • 3 starch
Carb Choices: 4

Zucchini, rich in the antioxidant glutathione, boosts the body's immune system and helps detoxify chemicals that can build up in the liver.

Quick Cream of Broccoli Soup

EASY • DO AHEAD • FREEZE   *Serves: 6*

16-ounce package frozen chopped broccoli, thawed and drained	**2 cups pre-cooked potato cubes**
3 cups nonfat chicken broth	**1 tablespoon onion powder**
1½ cups nonfat evaporated skim milk	**1 tablespoon celery flakes**
	1½ teaspoons minced garlic
	⅛ teaspoon cayenne

Set aside 1 cup of chopped broccoli. Combine the remaining ingredients in a large soup pot and bring to a boil over medium-high heat. Reduce heat to low, cover, and simmer for 30 to 45 minutes, stirring occasionally. Remove the soup from the heat and cool for 5 to 10 minutes. Working in batches, process the mixture in a food processor or blender until smooth. Pour the back into the pot; add the reserved broccoli and cook over medium heat until heated through. Soup can be frozen for up to 1 month.

Nutrition per serving: Calories 132 • Fat 0.5g • Carbohydrates 24g • Protein 10g • Cholesterol 3mg • Dietary fiber 4g • Sodium 486mg

Exchanges: 1 vegetable • 1 starch • ½ milk

Carb Choices: 2

Could you be one of these? Nearly one-third of Americans with high blood pressure don't know they have it.

Southwest Stew

EASY • DO AHEAD • FREEZE   *Serves:* 6

1½ pounds extra-lean ground
  beef
1 teaspoon garlic powder
1 cup frozen pepper stir-fry mix
16-ounce can black beans, rinsed
  and drained
11-ounce can corn kernels,
  drained

4-ounce can diced green chiles
¼ cup plus 2 tablespoons instant
  minced onion
2¼ cups water, divided
1½ teaspoons chili powder
½ teaspoon dried oregano
¼ teaspoon cayenne
1 tablespoon cornstarch

Spray a large pot or Dutch oven with cooking spray; add the ground beef, sprinkle with garlic powder, and cook, stirring frequently, for 5 to 6 minutes. Add the pepper stir-fry mix, black beans, corn kernels, green chiles, onions, 2 cups of the water, chili powder, oregano, and cayenne to the beef; bring to a boil over high heat. Immediately reduce heat to low, cover, and simmer for 10 minutes. Combine the remaining ¼ cup of water and cornstarch in a small bowl; mix until smooth. Stir the cornstarch mixture into the stew and cook over medium heat, stirring constantly, until thickened.

Nutrition per serving: Calories 287 • Fat 4.9g • Carbohydrates 31g • Protein 28g •
  Cholesterol 61mg • Dietary fiber 4g • Sodium 524mg
Exchanges: 2½ lean meat • 1½ starch • 1 vegetable
Carb Choices: 2

Lean red meat is an excellent source of zinc, a mineral that helps prevent acne-related skin breakouts.

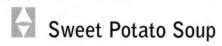 # Sweet Potato Soup

EASY • DO AHEAD   *Serves: 8*

2½ pounds sweet potatoes, peeled and cut into
  ½-inch slices
5 cups nonfat chicken or vegetable broth
2 cups sliced green onions
Pepper to taste

Place the potatoes in a large shallow baking dish; sprinkle with water and microwave on high heat for 10 to 12 minutes, until tender. Combine the 2½ cups of the broth and the green onions in a large soup pot; bring to a boil over high heat. Reduce the heat to low and simmer for 10 to 12 minutes. Remove from the stove top and cool for 10 minutes. Working in several batches, combine the broth and potatoes in a food processor or blender and process until smooth. Return the mixture to the soup pot. Add the remaining 2½ cups of broth; bring to a boil over medium-high heat, stirring frequently. Reduce heat to low and simmer for 20 to 30 minutes. Season with pepper to taste. Soup can be served hot or cold.

Nutrition per serving: Calories 158 • Fat 0.4g • Carbohydrates 35g • Protein 4g •
  Cholesterol 0mg • Dietary fiber 4g • Sodium 503mg
Exchanges: 2 starch
Carb Choices: 2

Sweet potatoes, baking potatoes, dried apricots, black currants, celery, fennel, green leafy vegetables, parsley, artichokes, and legumes are all high in potassium, which helps regulate blood pressure by enabling the body to dispose of more sodium.

Main Dish Meals

Baked Salmon Patties

EASY • DO AHEAD • FREEZE

Serves: 4

2 6½ ounce cans salmon,
  drained
1 cup Corn Flake crumbs, divided
1 tablespoon nonfat sour cream
2 tablespoons lemon juice

2 egg whites
½ teaspoon onion powder
½ teaspoon mustard
¾ teaspoon garlic powder

Preheat the oven to 350 degrees. Line a baking sheet with foil and spray with cooking spray. Combine the salmon, ¼ cup Corn Flake crumbs, sour cream, lemon juice, egg whites, onion powder, and mustard in a medium bowl; mix until the ingredients are blended. Shape into 4 patties. Combine the remaining ¾ cup of crumbs and garlic powder in a zip-top bag; shake until mixed. Place the salmon patties in the bag (one at a time) and gently shake until coated with crumb mixture. Place the breaded patties on the baking sheet. Bake for 20 to 25 minutes, until lightly browned and crisp.

Nutrition per serving: Calories 226 • Fat 5g • Carbohydrates 18g • Protein 24g •
  Cholesterol 36mg • Dietary fiber 0g • Sodium 727mg
Exchanges: 3 lean meat • 1 starch
Carb Choices: 1

Omega-rich fish including salmon, white albacore tuna, rainbow trout, anchovies, sardines, and mackerel not only lower the risk of heart attack deaths, but may also help treat depression, Crohn's disease, and some forms of arthritis.

Bean and Cheese Burrito

EASY · DO AHEAD   *Serves: 4*

2 cups nonfat refried beans
2 cups chunky-style salsa,
  divided
2 cups nonfat shredded cheddar
  cheese, divided
¼ cup chopped green onions
¼ cup diced green chiles,
  drained

¼ teaspoon ground cumin
4 10-inch low-fat flour tortillas
  (whole-wheat if available)
Nonfat sour cream, optional
Salsa, optional

Preheat the oven to 350 degrees. Spray a 9x13-inch baking dish with cooking spray. Spread ¾ cup of the salsa on the bottom of the baking dish. Combine the beans, ¾ cup of salsa, 1 cup of the cheese, green onions, green chiles, and cumin in a medium bowl and mix well. Spoon ⅓ to ½ cup of the bean mixture down the center of each tortilla. Roll the tortillas and place them seam-side down in the baking dish. Top with the remaining cup of cheese and ½ cup of salsa. Bake for 25 to 30 minutes. Serve the burritos with nonfat sour cream and salsa, if desired.

Nutrition per serving: Calories 380 · Fat 0.9g · Carbohydrates 58g · Protein 29g ·
  Cholesterol 0mg · Dietary fiber 7g · Sodium 2,163mg
Exchanges: 2 very lean meat · 3 starch · 2 vegetable ·
Carb Choices: 4

Adding half a cup of salsa to any meal is a simple way to boost your daily intake of vegetables.

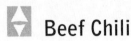 **Beef Chili**

EASY • DO AHEAD • FREEZE   *Serves: 4*

½ pound extra-lean ground beef, crumbled

2 tablespoons onion powder

1½ tablespoons dried sweet pepper flakes

1 teaspoon garlic powder

2 tablespoons plus 1 teaspoon chili powder

2 teaspoons unsweetened cocoa powder

14½-ounce can nonfat beef broth

14½-ounce can diced tomatoes with green chiles, undrained

1 cup water

15-ounce can chili beans, drained

1 cup canned corn kernels, drained

⅛ teaspoon cayenne

Spray a large nonstick skillet with cooking spray; place on a stove top and heat over medium-high heat until hot. Add the beef, onion powder, pepper flakes, and garlic powder; cook, stirring frequently, until the beef is browned and cooked through. Drain the meat in the colander. Spray a skillet again with cooking spray. Return the beef to the skillet; add the chili powder and cocoa powder and mix well. Add the broth, tomatoes, and water; bring to a boil over high heat. Cover the pan, reduce heat to low and simmer for 15 to 20 minutes. Uncover; stir in the beans, corn, and cayenne. Cook for 5 to 7 minutes over medium heat to heat through.

Nutrition per serving: Calories 239 • Fat 3.9g • Carbohydrates 31g • Protein 20g • Cholesterol 30mg • Dietary fiber 2g • Sodium 1,094 mg

Exchanges: 2 lean meat • 2 vegetable • 2 starch

Carb Choices: 2

Reduce fat when cooking ground beef by draining in a colander lined with paper towels.

Bountiful Burger

EASY • DO AHEAD • FREEZE   *Serves: 4*

⅓ cup uncooked bulgur

½ cup boiling water

¾ pound extra-lean ground beef
  or turkey

½ teaspoon minced garlic

¾ cup shredded zucchini

2 teaspoons steak sauce

¾ teaspoon Mrs. Dash seasoning

½ teaspoon ground pepper

2 whole-wheat buns, cut in half

Lettuce leaves, optional

Red onion slices, optional

Sliced tomato, optional

Sliced pickles, optional

Mustard, optional

Ketchup, optional

Nonfat ranch salad dressing,
  optional

Add the bulgur to the boiling water. Let stand for 30 minutes, until the liquid is absorbed and the bulgur is tender. Combine the cooked bulgur with the ground beef or turkey, garlic, zucchini, steak sauce, Mrs. Dash, and pepper. Shape into 4 half-inch thick patties. Preheat the broiler. Line a baking sheet with foil and spray with cooking spray. Arrange the patties in a single layer; cook for 5 to 6 minutes per side until cooked through. Place half a whole-wheat bun on each plate, top with a burger, and garnish as desired.

Nutrition per serving: Calories 210 • Fat 4.7g • Carbohydrates 20g • Protein 19g •
  Cholesterol 46mg • Dietary fiber 4g • Sodium 168mg
Exchanges: 2 lean meat • 1 starch • 1 vegetable
Carb Choices: 1

According to information provided by the USDA's Food Safety and Inspection Service and the National Turkey Foundation, a poultry product labeled "ground" may contain whole muscle material such as drumstick, thighs, neck, etc., with skin and adhering fat. On the other hand, a package labeled "ground turkey meat" only consists of ground muscle meat without the skin. The leanest type of ground poultry is ground turkey breast meat without the skin.

GREAT BURGER ADD-ONS

Reuben Burger: Top the burger with 1 slice (1 ounce) of nonfat Swiss cheese and broil for 30 seconds until melted. Spoon ¼ cup sauerkraut on top and serve.

Chili Burger: Top each burger with ¼ cup nonfat vegtarian canned chili with or without beans (heat in microwave on high 1 to 1½ minutes) and sprinkle with 1 to 2 tablespoons nonfat cheddar cheese. Garnish with chopped green onions as desired.

Cheeseburger: Top each burger with 1 slice (1 ounce) of nonfat cheese (American, Swiss, cheddar, mozzarella) and place under the broiler about 30 seconds, until melted. Garnish as desired.

Chicken and Bean Tostadas

EASY   *Serves: 4*

4 large low-fat flour tortillas
½ cup nonfat refried beans
½ cup chunky-style salsa
12-ounce package cooked
  chicken breast cuts,
  chopped fine
½ cup diced red onions
1 cup nonfat shredded cheddar
  cheese

½ cup nonfat sour cream,
  optional
2 cups shredded lettuce, optional
1½ cups chopped tomatoes,
  optional
Salsa, optional

Preheat the oven to 450 degrees. Line a baking sheet with foil and spray with cooking spray. Arrange the tortillas on the baking sheet; spread each tortilla with 2 tablespoons of refried beans. Layer the salsa, chicken, onions, and cheese on the tortilla. Place the baking sheet in the oven; bake for 10 to 12 minutes, until the cheese is melted. Turn on the broiler; broil for 30 to 45 seconds, until lightly browned on top. Serve tostadas with remaining optional ingredients and extra salsa.

Nutrition per serving: Calories 344 · Fat 4.2g · Carbohydrates 35g · Protein 38g · Cholesterol 64 mg · Dietary fiber 3 g · Sodium 955mg
Exchanges: 2 starch · 4½ lean meat · 1 vegetable
Carb Choices: 2

Limit choices at mealtimes. A 2001 study published in *Psychological Bulletin* found that when a variety of foods were available during a meal (i.e., buffet table), people ate as much as 44 percent more than those with only one food choice. While eating one food is not recommended because it will not provide proper nutrients, limiting the variety of food choices can cut caloric intake.

Chicken and Rice Ratatouille

EASY ▪ DO AHEAD ▪ FREEZE   *Serves: 4*

1 tablespoon nonfat chicken or
  vegetable broth
1 zucchini, unpeeled and
  sliced thin
1 yellow squash, unpeeled and
  sliced thin
1 small eggplant, peeled and cut
  into 1 inch cubes
1 medium onion, peeled and
  sliced thin
½ pound fresh sliced
  mushrooms

1 green bell pepper, cored, seeded,
  and cut into 1-inch pieces
15½-ounce can diced tomatoes,
  lightly drained
½ teaspoon garlic powder
1½ teaspoons Italian seasoning
Pepper to taste
12 ounces cooked and cubed
  chicken breast cuts
2 cups cooked brown rice

Spray a large nonstick skillet with cooking spray; add the broth and heat over medium-high heat. Add the zucchini, squash, eggplant, onion, mushrooms, and bell pepper; cook, stirring frequently for 12 to 15 minutes. Add the tomatoes, garlic powder, Italian seasoning, and pepper; bring to a boil over high heat. Reduce heat to low and simmer for 5 minutes. Add the chicken; heat through and serve over brown rice.

Nutrition per serving: Calories 318 • Fat 5 g • Carbohydrates 39g • Protein 29g •
  Cholesterol 64 mg • Dietary fiber 4g • Sodium 235 mg
Exchanges: 2 vegetable • 2 lean meat • 2 starch
Carb Choices: 3

Storing onions: Onions will keep about ten days in a well-ventilated, cool, dry place. Avoid storing in plastic bags or refrigerating as the humidity in these places makes onions break down. You can chop onions and freeze them, tightly wrapped, for up to three months.

Chicken-Fried Rice

EASY   *Serves: 4*

2 tablespoons nonfat chicken
  broth
2 cups cooked rice
½ cup frozen diced carrots,
  thawed and drained
½ cup frozen baby peas, slightly
  thawed

⅓ cup chopped green onions
¾ teaspoon minced garlic
2 tablespoons low-sodium
  soy sauce
12-ounce package cooked and
  cubed chicken breast cuts

Spray a large nonstick skillet with cooking spray; add the broth and heat over medium-high heat. Add the rice, carrots, peas, onions, and minced garlic; cook for 1 to 2 minutes. Drizzle the soy sauce over the rice mixture; toss lightly to mix. Stir in the chicken and heat through. Serve immediately.

Nutrition per serving: Calories 290 • Fat 4g • Carbohydrates 34g • Protein 28g •
  Cholesterol 64mg • Dietary fiber 2g • Sodium 381mg
Exchanges: 2 starch • 1 vegetable • 3 very lean meat
Carb Choices: 2

Unopened bottles of soy sauce can be safely stored for up to three years; once the bottle has been opened, use within nine months.

Cod Fillets with Dijon Sauce

EASY • DO AHEAD   *Serves: 4*

1½ pounds cod fillets
4½ tablespoons nonfat
  mayonnaise
1½ tablespoons Dijon mustard
¾ tablespoon prepared
  horseradish

½ teaspoon celery seed
2 tablespoons seasoned bread
  crumbs

Preheat the oven to 350 degrees. Line a baking sheet with foil and spray with cooking spray. Arrange the cod fillets in a single layer; fold ends under so the fillets are all the same thickness. Combine the mayonnaise, mustard, horseradish, and celery seed in a small bowl; mix well and spread evenly over the fish. Sprinkle with the bread crumbs; spray lightly with cooking spray. Bake the fish for 15 to 20 minutes, until lightly browned and fish flakes easily with a fork.

Nutrition per serving: Calories 172 • Fat 1.6g • Carbohydrates 6g • Protein 31g •
  Cholesterol 62mg • Dietary fiber 0g • Sodium 340 mg
Exchanges: 4 very lean meat • ½ other carb
Carb Choices: 0

Top choice seasonings for fish and seafood include lemon juice, Dijon mustard, cayenne, cumin, marjoram, and mint.

Crusted Baked Salmon

EASY   *Serves: 4*

2 tablespoons Butter Buds
1 to 2 tablespoons water
2½ tablespoons Dijon mustard
1½ tablespoons honey
¼ cup Corn Flake crumbs

2 tablespoons finely chopped
pecans
1 pound salmon fillets
Lemon wedges for garnish,
optional

Combine the Butter Buds and water in a small bowl; mix until dissolved. Add the mustard and honey to the Butter Buds and mix well. Combine the Corn Flake crumbs and pecans in a zip-top bag; shake to mix. Preheat the oven to 450 degrees. Line a baking sheet with foil and spray with cooking spray. Arrange the salmon fillets on the baking sheet; brush on both sides with honey-mustard mixture. Sprinkle the Corn Flake crumb mixture over the top; turn and coat on the other side. Bake the salmon for 10 minutes per inch of thickness, or until the fish flakes easily with a fork. Garnish with lemon wedges, if desired.

Nutrition per serving: Calories 230 · Fat 7.1g · Carbohydrates 17g · Protein 23g ·
    Cholesterol 59mg · Dietary fiber <1g · Sodium 277mg
Exchanges: 3 lean meat · 1 other carb
Carb Choices: 1

Researchers at Harvard University found that when nuts were substituted for other sources of dietary fat, the risk of heart disease dropped by 45 percent.

Dill Salmon with Vegetables

EASY • DO AHEAD   *Serves: 4*

¼ cup white wine vinegar	1 large onion, thinly sliced
¼ teaspoon Dijon mustard	½ cup nonfat cottage cheese
1¼ teaspoons dried dill, divided	¼ cup nonfat mayonnaise
1½ pounds salmon fillets	¼ cup skim milk
1 large bell pepper, thinly sliced	1 tablespoon lemon juice
1 large tomato, thinly sliced	½ teaspoon minced garlic

Combine the vinegar, mustard, and ¼ teaspoon of the dill in a small bowl; mix well. Line a baking sheet with foil and spray with cooking spray. Arrange the salmon fillets in a single layer on the baking sheet; pour the sauce over the fish and coat on both sides. Let the fish marinate 5 to 10 minutes. Preheat the oven to 375 degrees. Arrange the pepper, tomato, and onion slices on the salmon; cover tightly with foil and bake for 15 to 20 minutes, until the fish flakes easily with a fork and the vegetables are softened. While the fish is cooking, combine the cottage cheese, mayonnaise, milk, lemon juice, garlic, and remaining 1 teaspoon of dill in a food processor or blender and puree until smooth and creamy. Cover and refrigerate until ready to serve.

Nutrition per serving: Calories 254 • Fat 6.1g • Carbohydrates 12g • Protein 37g • Cholesterol 89mg • Dietary fiber 2g • Sodium 261mg

Exchanges: 3 lean meat • 1 vegetable • ½ other carb

Carb Choices: 1

Researchers at Brigham and Women's Hospital and Harvard Medical School found that eating at least one serving of fish each week can cut your risk of dying from a heart-related disease in half. This is a case where fatter may be better; fish rich in omega-3 fats include salmon, rainbow trout, and swordfish.

Grilled Chicken Breasts with Papaya Salsa

EASY · DO AHEAD   *Serves: 4*

1 pound ripe papaya, peeled and diced	¼ cup fresh lime juice
2 tablespoons diced green chiles, drained	2 tablespoons minced cilantro
3 kiwifruits, peeled and diced	1 pound boneless, skinless chicken breasts
½ teaspoon minced garlic	1½ teaspoons onion powder
¼ cup diced red onion	¾ teaspoon garlic powder

Combine the papaya, green chiles, kiwi, minced garlic, red onion, lime juice, and cilantro in a medium bowl; mix well. Cover and refrigerate for at least 6 hours, or overnight. Preheat the broiler. Line a broiler pan with foil and spray with cooking spray. Arrange chicken breasts in a single layer on the pan; sprinkle on both sides with onion and garlic powder. Broil for 8 to 10 minutes per side until completely cooked through. Serve broiled chicken with papaya salsa.

Nutrition per serving: Calories 204 • Fat 1.4g • Carbohydrates 23g • Protein 24g •
    Cholesterol 0mg • Dietary fiber 3g • Sodium 600mg
Exchanges: 1 fruit • 2 vegetable • 3 very lean meat
Carb Choices: 2

Mangoes and papayas contain beta-cryptoxanthin, a phytochemical that may reduce the risk of certain types of cancer.

Grilled Chicken with Sweet Potato Slices

EASY   *Serves: 4*

¾ cup plus 1½ tablespoons
   nonfat chicken broth, divided
1 pound boneless, skinless
   chicken breasts, cut into
   ¼-inch thick slices
1 tablespoon onion powder
¾ cup apple cider

1½ teaspoons cornstarch
2 teaspoons minced garlic
¾ pound sweet potatoes, peeled
   and cut into ½-inch thick
   slices
2 apples, cored and cut into
   ½-inch wedges

Spray a large nonstick skillet with cooking spray; add 1½ tablespoons of the chicken broth and heat over medium-high heat. Add the chicken slices; sprinkle with onion powder and cook, stirring frequently, for 2 to 3 minutes per side. Remove the skillet from the heat and set aside. Combine the cider and cornstarch in a small bowl; mix until completely smooth. Add the cider mixture, remaining ¾ cup of broth, garlic, sweet potatoes, and apples to the skillet with the chicken. Bring to a boil over medium-high heat. Cover, reduce heat, and cook for 30 to 35 minutes until the potatoes and apples are cooked through.

Nutrition per serving: Calories 273 · Fat 1.5g · Carbohydrates 39g · Protein 24g ·
   Cholesterol 0mg · Dietary fiber 4g · Sodium 718mg
Exchanges: 2½ very lean meat · 1 fruit · 1½ starch
Carb Choices: 3

Researchers at the University of California at Davis found that drinking twelve ounces of apple juice or eating two whole apples a day can reduce the oxidation of LDL cholesterol. Packed with antioxidants, potassium, fiber, and other key nutrients, the phytochemicals in apples can help cut the risk of death from heart disease or stroke in half.

Grilled Halibut with Orange Salsa

EASY • DO AHEAD   *Serves: 4*

1 cup canned diced tomatoes,
    drained well
2 oranges, peeled, seeded,
    and diced
3 tablespoons diced red onion
1 teaspoon dried cilantro
1½ tablespoons orange juice

1¼ teaspoons balsamic vinegar
1½ teaspoons minced garlic
½ teaspoon ground ginger
⅛ teaspoon cayenne
1½ pounds halibut steaks, about
    1-inch thick
½ cup low-sodium teriyaki sauce

Combine the diced tomatoes, oranges, red onion, cilantro, orange juice, vinegar, minced garlic, ginger, and cayenne in a medium bowl; toss and mix well. Cover and refrigerate for at least 1 hour. Place the halibut steaks in a shallow dish; pour the teriyaki sauce over the top and turn to coat. Cover and refrigerate for 1½ to 2 hours, turning several times. Preheat the broiler. Line a broiler pan with foil and spray with cooking spray. Remove the fish from the marinade and place on the broiler pan. Broil 4 to 6 minutes; turn the fish over and broil for 4 to 6 minutes, until the fish flakes easily with a fork and the center is opaque. Top the halibut with salsa and serve.

Nutrition per serving: Calories 267 • Fat 4.1g • Carbohydrates 18g • Protein 38g •
    Cholesterol 54 mg • Dietary fiber 2g • Sodium 831mg
Exchanges: 1 vegetable • 5 very lean meat • 1 other carb
Carb Choices: 1

According to a twelve-year study reported in the *Annals of Internal Medicine* (February 5, 2002), a diet rich in red meat, processed meat, french fries, high-fat dairy foods, refined grains, and sweets increases diabetes risk to 60 percent above average, twice the risk of those eating a diet rich in vegetables, fruits, whole grains, fish, and poultry. The same study showed that following the healthier diet can reduce the risk of diabetes by 20 percent below average.

Heart-Healthy Stuffed Cabbage

AVERAGE • DO AHEAD • FREEZE   *Serves: 4*

1 head cabbage, cored and rinsed	1 small onion, peeled and sliced
1 pound extra-lean ground turkey	½ cup packaged shredded cabbage
1 tablespoon onion powder	¾ cup shredded carrots
½ cup bread crumbs	1 tablespoon lemon juice
1¼ cups water, divided	2 tablespoons brown sugar
⅛ teaspoon pepper	1 tablespoon cornstarch
15½-ounce can diced tomatoes, drained and liquid reserved	

Remove 8 outer leaves from the cabbage; place them in a saucepan, cover with boiling water, and simmer over medium-low heat for 5 minutes, until softened. Drain the cabbage leaves in a colander and pat dry with paper towels. Spray a large nonstick skillet with cooking spray; add the turkey and onion powder. Cook, stirring frequently, until browned and cooked through. Remove the turkey from the skillet and place in a medium mixing bowl; add the bread crumbs, ¼ cup of the water, and pepper and mix well. Add ½ cup of the reserved tomato liquid to the turkey mixture; mix well. Spray the skillet again with cooking spray. Spoon the turkey filling (about ¼ to ⅓ cup) onto the cooked cabbage leaves; wrap the leaf around the filling and place seam-side down in the skillet. Add the drained tomatoes, sliced onion, shredded cabbage, the remaining 1 cup of water, and carrots; cover the skillet and cook over medium-low heat for 55 to 60 minutes, basting several times. Remove the cabbage rolls from the skillet; set aside and keep warm. Combine the lemon juice, brown sugar, and cornstarch in a small bowl; mix until the sugar and cornstarch are dissolved and the mixture is thickened. Add to the skillet (with vegetables); cook, stirring constantly, until the sauce thickens. Serve sauce over warm cabbage rolls.

Nutrition per serving: Calories 238 • Fat 2.2g • Carbohydrates 27g • Protein 30g • Cholesterol 46g • Dietary fiber 4g • Sodium 318mg

Exchanges: 3 very lean meat • 4 vegetable • ½ other carb

Carb Choices: 2

> Ground poultry dishes should always be cooked to 165 degrees internal temperature.

Italian Beef Pita Pockets

EASY • DO AHEAD   *Serves:* 6

1 pound extra-lean ground beef
1 tablespoon plus ¾ teaspoon
   onion powder, divided
3 teaspoons garlic powder, divided
2 teaspoons sweet dried pepper
   flakes
½ cup plus 2 tablespoons low-
   sodium soy sauce, divided
¼ cup Worcestershire sauce,
   divided

½ teaspoon cumin
1 teaspoon Italian seasoning, divided
¼ cup white vinegar
3 whole-wheat pita pockets, cut
   in half
1½ cups shredded lettuce
¾ cup canned diced tomatoes with
   garlic and onions, drained well
¾ cup nonfat shredded mozzarella
   cheese

Spray a large nonstick skillet with cooking spray; add the ground beef, 1 table-spoon of the onion powder, 2 teaspoons of the garlic powder, and pepper flakes to the skillet. Cook, stirring frequently, until the beef is browned and cooked through. Stir in 2 tablespoons of the soy sauce, 2 tablespoons of the Worcester-shire sauce, the remaining ½ teaspoon of garlic powder, cumin, and ½ teaspoon of the Italian seasoning and mix well. Cook over medium-low heat for 10 to 15 minutes. Combine the remaining ½ cup of soy sauce, 2 tablespoons Worcester-shire sauce, vinegar, ¾ teaspoon of onion powder, and ½ teaspoon of garlic powder in a small saucepan; bring to a boil over high heat. Reduce the heat to low and simmer for 5 to 10 minutes. Fill the pita pockets with the beef mixture; top with the sauce. Garnish with shredded lettuce, diced tomatoes, and shred-ded cheese, as desired.

Nutrition per serving: Calories 204 • Fat 3.4g • Carbohydrates 17g • Protein 23g •
   Dietary fiber 1g • Sodium 1,323mg
Exchanges: 2 lean meat • 1 starch • 1 vegetable
Carb Choices: 1

Fresh, cooked, or powdered garlic all have the cardio-protective qualities. Garlic lowers total cholesterol, improves blood pressure, and is a powerful antioxidant.

Lahvosh Vegetarian Pizza

EASY • DO AHEAD   *Serves: 6*

1½ cups broccoli florets, cut
  into small pieces
1 cup cauliflower florets, sliced
½ cup diced asparagus
1 cup nonfat pizza sauce
1 large whole-wheat lahvosh
  cracker

2 cups nonfat shredded
  mozzarella cheese, divided
1 cup canned diced tomatoes,
  drained well
½ cup sliced mushrooms
1 cup bell pepper strips
¼ cup nonfat Parmesan cheese

Preheat the oven to 425 degrees. Line a baking sheet or pizza pan with foil and spray with cooking spray. Combine the broccoli, cauliflower, and asparagus in a shallow glass dish; sprinkle with water and microwave on high for 3 to 5 minutes, until tender crisp. Spread the pizza sauce on the lahvosh; top with 1½ cups of the mozzarella cheese. Arrange the cooked broccoli, cauliflower, and asparagus. Add the diced tomatoes, sliced mushrooms, and pepper strips; top with the remaining ½ cup of mozzarella and the Parmesan cheese. Bake 12 to 15 minutes, until the cheese is melted and lightly browned.

Nutrition per serving: Calories 126 • Fat 0.4g • Carbohydrates 13g • Protein 17g •
  Cholesterol 0mg • Dietary fiber 3g • Sodium 483mg
Exchanges: ½ starch • 2 vegetable • 1½ very lean meat
Carb Choices: 1

Don't rely on color to tell a whole grain from a refined one. Some brown foods are as refined as white. Instead, look for the word "whole" in the front of the grain on the package ingredients list.

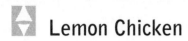 # Lemon Chicken

EASY • DO AHEAD   *Serves: 4*

4 to 5 fresh lemons	1½ pounds boneless, skinless
2 tablespoons white wine vinegar	chicken breasts
1 tablespoon onion powder	1 teaspoon garlic powder
1 teaspoon dried Italian	Pepper to taste
seasoning	

Squeeze the juice from the lemons; reserve ½ cup juice. Peel the lemons; slice and reserve ½ cup of the fresh peel. Combine the lemon juice, lemon peel, vinegar, onion powder, and Italian seasoning in a small bowl. Spray a 9x13-inch baking dish with cooking spray; arrange the chicken breasts in the dish. Sprinkle chicken on both sides with garlic powder. Pour the lemon sauce over the chicken, cover, and refrigerate for at least 6 hours or overnight. Turn the chicken several times while marinating. Preheat the oven to 325 degrees. Bake, covered, for 30 minutes; remove the cover, sprinkle with pepper, and bake for 25 to 30 minutes, until cooked through.

Nutrition per serving: Calories 182 • Fat 1.5g • Carbohydrates 5g • Protein 34g • Cholesterol 0mg • Dietary fiber 0g • Sodium 814mg
Exchanges: 5 very lean meat
Carb Choices: 0

Shop the perimeter of the grocery store to stay focused on fresh, healthy foods found in the produce, dairy, fish, and meat sections, while avoiding the highly processed foods and snacks in the inner aisles.

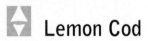 Lemon Cod

EASY   *Serves: 4*

1 pound cod fillets   **1 tablespoon lemon juice**
½ teaspoon garlic powder   **1 teaspoon celery seed**
½ cup nonfat mayonnaise   **½ teaspoon grated lemon peel**

Preheat the grill or broiler on medium-high heat. If broiling, line a baking sheet with foil and spray with cooking spray. Sprinkle the cod with garlic powder on both sides and place on the baking sheet. Combine the remaining ingredients in a small bowl. Brush the fish with half the mayonnaise-lemon mixture; broil or grill for 5 minutes. Carefully turn the fish over; brush with the remaining sauce and broil or grill for 5 minutes, until the fish flakes easily with a fork.

Nutrition per serving: Calories 118 • Fat 0.8g • Carbohydrates 5g • Protein 20g •
   Cholesterol 49mg • Dietary fiber 0g • Sodium 272mg
Exchanges: 3 very lean meat • ½ other carb
Carb Choices: 0

What you eat, along with regular exercise, can keep blood cholesterol levels in check and reduce your risk of heart disease. Since our bodies produce cholesterol, doctors recommend consuming no more than 300 milligrams a day of this fatty substance from dietary sources. Five foods that contribute to steady blood cholesterol levels include soy, salmon, garlic, oats, and plant foods.

Lentil Pasta with Diced Tomatoes

AVERAGE *Serves: 4*

2 cups water
½ cup dry red lentils, sorted
and rinsed
¼ teaspoon crushed bay leaf
28-ounce can diced tomatoes,
drained
½ teaspoon minced garlic

½ teaspoon red pepper flakes
2 cups ditalini or orzo, cooked
according to package
directions
2 tablespoons nonfat Parmesan
cheese

Pour the water into a large saucepan; bring to a boil over high heat. Add the lentils and bay leaf; reduce the heat to medium and cook, stirring occasionally, until the lentils are tender (about 15 to 20 minutes). Drain well. Spray a large nonstick skillet with cooking spray. Add the diced tomatoes, garlic, and pepper flakes; cook over medium heat, stirring frequently, until most of the liquid is absorbed. Stir in the cooked lentils. Add the cooked pasta; toss lightly and sprinkle with cheese. Serve immediately.

Nutrition per serving: Calories 321 · Fat 1.5g · Carbohydrates 63g · Protein 16g ·
   Cholesterol 0mg · Dietary fiber 2g · Sodium 354mg
Exchanges: 3½ starch · 2 vegetable
Carb Choices: 4

Harvard Medical School researchers found that women who ate about 26 grams of fiber daily from fruits, vegetables, and whole grains lowered their risk of heart disease and heart attacks.

Linguine with Scallops

EASY   *Serves: 6*

12-ounce package linguine	**½ teaspoon red pepper flakes**
2 tablespoons white wine	**15½-ounce can crushed**
1½ pounds bay scallops	**tomatoes**
1 teaspoon minced garlic	**¾ cup nonfat Parmesan cheese,**
2 teaspoons dried parsley	**optional**
½ teaspoon dried oregano	

Cook the linguine according to package directions; drain and keep warm.
Spray a large nonstick skillet with cooking spray; add the wine and heat over
medium-high heat. Add the scallops; cook 2 to 3 minutes, until the scallops turn
white. Add the garlic; cook 1 to 2 minutes. Remove the scallops from the skillet and keep warm. Add the parsley, oregano, red pepper flakes, and tomatoes
to the skillet; cook over medium heat 5 to 6 minutes, until heated through. Toss
the pasta, scallops, and sauce in a bowl; serve with Parmesan cheese, if desired.

Nutrition per serving: Calories 328 • Fat 1.9g • Carbohydrates 48g • Protein 27g •
Cholesterol 37mg • Dietary fiber 1g • Sodium 307mg
Exchanges: 2 very lean meat • 3 starch • 1 vegetable
Carb Choices: 3

The iodine in scallops and other seafood is used to produce thyroid hormones that are key to revving up metabolism.

Main Meal Meat Loaf

EASY ▪ DO AHEAD ▪ FREEZE   *Serves: 6*

1½ pounds extra-lean ground
  beef
2 teaspoons onion powder
¾ cup quick-cooking oatmeal,
  uncooked
½ cup ketchup
2 tablespoons horseradish
2 tablespoons lemon juice

¼ cup egg substitute
1 tablespoon Worcestershire
  sauce
2 teaspoons chopped garlic
½ teaspoon dried basil
Pepper to taste

Preheat the oven to 350 degrees. Line a baking sheet with foil and spray with cooking spray. Combine all the ingredients in a large bowl and mix well. Shape the mixture into an 8-inch loaf. Bake for 50 to 55 minutes, until cooked through and no longer pink. Let the meat loaf stand for 5 minutes before slicing and serving.

Nutrition per serving: Calories 213 · Fat 5.2g · Carbohydrates 14g · Protein 24g ·
  Cholesterol 61mg · Dietary fiber <1g · Sodium 311mg
Exchanges: 2½ lean meat · 1 other carb
Carb Choices: 1

> The USDA classifies seven cuts of beef as lean: eye round, top round, round tip, top sirloin, bottom round, top loin, and tenderloin. If it has "round" or "loin" in its name, it's your healthiest bet on beef.

Orange Roughy Provençale

EASY • DO AHEAD   *Serves: 4*

¼ cup plus 1 tablespoon nonfat
  vegetable broth, divided
1½ cups frozen diced onion
28-ounce can diced tomatoes,
  drained
1 teaspoon minced garlic
1 bay leaf

¾ teaspoon dried thyme
¼ teaspoon pepper
1 pound orange roughy fillets
1 cup thinly sliced yellow squash
1 cup thinly sliced zucchini
1 cup bell pepper strips

Preheat the oven to 350 degrees. Spray a shallow baking dish with cooking spray. Spray a nonstick skillet with cooking spray; add 1 tablespoon of the vegetable broth and heat over medium-high heat. Add the onions; cook, stirring frequently, until softened. Add the drained tomatoes, garlic, bay leaf, remaining ¼ cup of vegetable broth, thyme, and pepper; reduce heat to medium-low, cover, and cook for 10 to 12 minutes, stirring occasionally. Place the fish fillets in the baking dish in a single layer. Place yellow squash, zucchini, and pepper slices around the fish; spoon the tomato sauce evenly over the fish and vegetables. Cover with heavy-duty foil and bake for 30 to 40 minutes, until the fish flakes easily with a fork.

Nutrition per serving: Calories 163 • Fat 1.1g • Carbohydrates 16g • Protein 20g •
  Cholesterol 23mg • Dietary fiber 3g • Sodium 457mg
Exchanges: 3 vegetable • 2 very lean meat
Carb Choices: 1

Fish fact: A fish fillet is a section of a full-size fish while a steak is a cross-section of the whole fish. Fillets generally come with the skin on, while steaks are usually thicker and skinless.

Pan-fried Mahimahi with Horseradish Sauce

EASY   *Serves: 4*

1 cup nonfat sour cream
2 teaspoons dried parsley
1 tablespoon prepared
  horseradish
1 tablespoon lemon juice
1 teaspoon Dijon mustard
Dash of cayenne

3 large egg whites, lightly beaten
2 tablespoons flour
¾ teaspoon dried basil
½ teaspoon dried oregano
¼ teaspoon pepper
1 pound mahimahi fillets

Combine the sour cream, parsley, horseradish, lemon juice, mustard, and cayenne in a small bowl; mix until smooth and creamy. Cover and refrigerate for 15 to 30 minutes. Place the egg whites in a shallow bowl and beat lightly. Combine the flour, basil, oregano, and pepper on a paper plate and mix well. Spray a nonstick skillet with cooking spray and heat over medium heat. Dip the fillets into the egg whites; dredge through the flour mixture. Cook for 5 minutes per side, until the fish flakes easily with a fork. Serve the fish with horseradish sauce.

Nutrition per serving: Calories 176 • Fat 1.2g • Carbohydrates 10g • Protein 28g •
   Cholesterol 81mg • Dietary fiber <1g • Sodium 254mg
Exchanges: 3½ very lean meat • ½ other carb
Carb Choices: 1

If you're trying to lose weight, make sure horseradish, mustard, and salsa are on your shopping list, advises recent guidelines on obesity from the National Heart, Lung, and Blood Institute (NHLBI). These condiments received high marks throughout the guidelines for their low-fat, high-flavor qualities.

Pineapple Chicken Packet

EASY • DO AHEAD   *Serves: 4*

16-ounce can pineapple chunks,   ¾ cup canned corn kernels,
   packed in juice, undrained   drained
1 pound boneless, skinless   ¾ cup chopped fresh cilantro
   chicken breasts, cut into   2 teaspoons chili powder
   1-inch slices   ⅛ teaspoon cayenne
¾ cup canned black beans,
   drained

Preheat the oven to 350 degrees. Drain the pineapple into a bowl, reserving the juice. Combine the chicken, pineapple, 3 tablespoons of pineapple juice, black beans, corn, cilantro, chili powder, and cayenne in a large bowl; toss to mix. Tear off four 10-inch pieces of heavy-duty foil and spray with cooking spray; divide the chicken mixture among foil sheets. Wrap foil around chicken mixture, leaving room at the top, and seal tightly. Place foil packets on a baking sheet; bake for 35 to 40 minutes, until the chicken is cooked through. If desired, serve over cooked rice (½ cup per serving).

Nutrition per serving: Calories 252 • Fat 1.8g • Carbohydrates 33g • Protein 27g •
  Cholesterol 0mg • Dietary fiber 4g • Sodium 834mg
Exchanges: 1 starch • 1 fruit • 3 very lean meat
Carb Choices: 2

> Canned and fresh pineapple contain identical nutritional value; both are fat-free, cholesterol-free, and low in sodium, while excellent sources of vitamin C, iron, and fiber.

Salmon Loaf with Dijon Sauce

EASY · DO AHEAD   *Serves: 8*

2 15½-ounce cans salmon,
  drained well
½ cup shredded zucchini
½ cup shredded carrots
1 cup quick-cooking oatmeal,
  uncooked
1¾ cup nonfat sour cream,
  divided
1 teaspoon onion powder

1 egg white
¼ cup egg substitute
2 tablespoons chopped
  pimientos
2 tablespoons Dijon mustard,
  divided
¼ teaspoon pepper
¾ cup frozen peas, thawed
1 teaspoon celery seed

Preheat the oven to 350 degrees. Spray an 8- or 9-inch loaf pan with cooking spray. Combine the salmon, zucchini, carrots, oatmeal, 1 cup of the sour cream, onion powder, egg white, egg substitute, pimientos, 1 tablespoon of the Dijon mustard, and pepper in a large bowl; mix lightly until the ingredients are well mixed. Combine the remaining 1 tablespoon of Dijon mustard, ¾ cup of sour cream, peas, and celery seed in a small bowl; mix well. Cover and refrigerate while the salmon loaf is baking. Press the salmon mixture into the loaf pan; bake for 55 to 60 minutes, until lightly browned. Let the salmon loaf stand for 5 minutes before slicing and serving with Dijon sauce.

Nutrition per serving: Calories 258 · Fat 7.1g · Carbohydrates 15g · Protein 30g ·
  Cholesterol 43mg · Dietary fiber 1g · Sodium 660mg
Exchanges: 3 lean meat · 1 vegetable · ½ starch · ½ other carb
Carb Choices: 1

Fish fact: When cooking fish in foil or sauce, add 5 minutes to the total cooking time.

Simple Seafood Bake

EASY • DO AHEAD   *Serves: 4*

1 pound mahimahi fillets   **½ teaspoon celery seed**
½ pound small shrimp, peeled   **¼ teaspoon pepper**
** and deveined**   **1 tablespoon lemon juice**
½ cup nonfat mayonnaise

Preheat the oven to 350 degrees. Spray a shallow baking dish with cooking spray; arrange the fish fillets in a single layer in the baking dish. Place the shrimp on top. Combine the mayonnaise, celery seed, pepper, and lemon juice in a small bowl; mix well. Spread the mayonnaise mixture over the fish; bake for 15 to 18 minutes, until the fish flakes easily with a fork.

Nutrition per serving: Calories 184 • Fat 2g • Carbohydrates 6g • Protein 33g • Cholesterol 168mg • Dietary fiber 0g • Sodium 407mg
Exchanges: ½ other carb • 4 very lean meat
Carb Choices: 0

Do not marinate shrimp for more than one hour; marinating longer than an hour will cause the shrimp to become soft and mushy.

Simply Stir-Fried with Brown Rice

AVERAGE   *Serves: 6*

½ cup plus 1½ tablespoons nonfat
  beef broth, divided
1½ teaspoons powdered ginger
1½ teaspoons minced garlic
1 pound boneless, skinless chicken
  breasts, cut into 2-inch strips
3 tablespoons low-sodium soy sauce
1 tablespoon cornstarch
16-ounce package frozen pepper
  stir-fry

10-ounce package frozen
  broccoli florets
10-ounce package frozen sliced
  carrots
1 cup sliced water chestnuts,
  drained
1 cup fresh bean sprouts
3 cups cooked brown rice

Combine 2 teaspoons of the beef broth, ginger, and garlic in a small bowl; blend until smooth. Pour the ginger sauce over the chicken strips, cover, and let stand 10 minutes. Combine ½ cup of the broth, soy sauce, and cornstarch in a small bowl; mix until smooth and set aside. Spray a large nonstick skillet with cooking spray; add the chicken and cook, stirring frequently for 5 to 6 minutes, until lightly browned and cooked through. Remove the chicken from the skillet and set aside. Add 2 teaspoons of the broth to the skillet; add the pepper stir-fry mix, broccoli, carrots, and water chestnuts; cook, stirring frequently, for 6 to 8 minutes, until the vegetables are tender crisp. Add the reserved soy sauce mixture, cooked chicken, and bean sprouts. Toss the mixture and cook, stirring constantly, for 2 to 3 minutes, until the sauce is thickened and heated through. Serve over cooked brown rice.

Nutrition per serving: Calories 265 • Fat 1.7g • Carbohydrates 40g • Protein 21g •
  Cholesterol 0mg • Dietary fiber 5g • Sodium 787mg
Exchanges: 2 very lean meat • 2 vegetable • 2 starch
Carb Choices: 3

Sprouts are full of natural vitamins, minerals, live enzymes, and amino acids. When they are sprouted and consumed in our digestive system, our bodies are able to absorb vital food factors that scientists believe can stimulate the body's immune system, thereby promoting better health.

Stir-Fry Chinese Chicken

EASY   *Serves: 4*

½ cup orange juice
1 teaspoon crushed garlic
¼ cup barbecue sauce
¼ cup Hoisin sauce
¼ teaspoon ground ginger

1 pound boneless, skinless
   chicken breasts, cut into
   1-inch cubes
1½ tablespoons nonfat chicken
   broth
2 cups cooked brown rice

Combine the orange juice, crushed garlic, barbecue sauce, Hoisin sauce, and ginger in a medium bowl; mix well. Add the chicken cubes to the sauce, cover, and marinate in the refrigerator for 1 to 2 hours, or overnight. Spray a large nonstick skillet with cooking spray; add the chicken broth and heat over medium-high heat. Add the marinated chicken to the skillet and cook, stirring frequently, for 7 to 8 minutes, until cooked through. Serve over cooked brown rice, if desired.

Nutrition per serving: Calories 276 · Fat 2.9g · Carbohydrates 34g · Protein 25g ·
   Cholesterol 0mg · Dietary fiber <1g · Sodium 864mg
Exchanges: 2 starch · ½ other carb · 2½ very lean meat
Carb Choices: 2

> For low-fat cooking, baste foods with wine, fruit juice, or marinade instead of pan drippings.

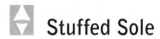

Stuffed Sole

EASY • DO AHEAD   *Serves: 4*

1 tablespoon nonfat chicken or
  vegetable broth
½ pound fresh sliced mushrooms
10-ounce package frozen
  chopped spinach, thawed and
  drained
¼ teaspoon Italian seasoning

½ teaspoon garlic powder
1½ pounds sole fillets, cut into
  4 pieces
1 tablespoon apple juice
1 cup nonfat shredded
  mozzarella cheese

Preheat the oven to 400 degrees. Spray a 10x6-inch baking dish with cooking spray. Spray a nonstick skillet with cooking spray; add the broth and heat over medium-high heat. Add the mushrooms to the skillet; cook, stirring frequently, for 2 to 3 minutes, until tender. Add the spinach; cook for 1 to 2 minutes, until heated. Remove the skillet from the heat; drain the liquid into the baking dish. Sprinkle the mushrooms and spinach with Italian seasoning and garlic powder and mix lightly. Divide the vegetable mixture evenly and spread down the center of each fillet. Roll the fillet around the filling and place seam-side down in the baking dish. Drizzle the apple juice over the fillets; sprinkle with the cheese. Bake for 15 to 20 minutes, until the cheese is melted and the fish flakes easily with a fork.

Nutrition per serving: Calories 220 • Fat 2.1g • Carbohydrates 7g • Protein 41g •
  Cholesterol 80mg • Dietary fiber 2g • Sodium 401mg
Exchanges: 2 vegetable • 5 very lean meat
Carb Choices: 0

Quick Tip: Cook individually "quick frozen" fish fillets without thawing by doubling the cooking time (about 16 to 20 minutes per inch of thickness of fish).

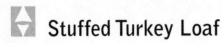

Stuffed Turkey Loaf

EASY • DO AHEAD • FREEZE   *Serves: 6*

1½ pounds 99 percent fat-free
   ground turkey
¾ teaspoon garlic powder
1½ teaspoons onion powder
1 cup quick-cooking oatmeal,
   uncooked
½ cup shredded zucchini

10-ounce package frozen
   chopped spinach, thawed
   and drained
¼ cup egg substitute
⅓ cup skim milk
1½ teaspoons Italian seasoning
2 tablespoons nonfat pasta sauce

Preheat the oven to 350 degrees. Line a baking sheet with foil and spray with cooking spray. Combine all the ingredients except the pasta sauce in a medium bowl and mix well. Shape the mixture into a loaf and place on a baking sheet. Brush the top with the pasta sauce. Bake for 50 to 55 minutes, until no longer pink and completely cooked through; let the turkey loaf stand for 5 minutes before slicing. Serve with additional pasta sauce, if desired.

Nutrition per serving: Calories 202 • Fat 2.5g • Carbohydrates 14g • Protein 32g •
   Cholesterol 46mg • Dietary fiber 2g • Sodium 174mg
Exchanges: ½ starch • 1 vegetable • 4 very lean meat
Carb Choices: 1

Oats, barley, and psyllium-enriched cereals lower heart-disease risk by adding cholesterol-fighting soluble fiber.

Turkey Cheese Burgers

EASY · DO AHEAD · FREEZE   *Serves: 6*

1 pound 99 percent fat-free
    ground turkey breast
1 cup quick-cooking oatmeal,
    uncooked
1 tablespoon onion powder
1 tablespoon dried sweet pepper
    flakes
¼ cup shredded carrots
¼ cup shredded zucchini
2 tablespoons barbecue sauce
2 tablespoons ketchup
1 teaspoon minced garlic

4 ounces nonfat American
    cheese slices
6 whole-wheat low-fat
    hamburger buns
Lettuce, optional
Sliced tomato, optional
Sliced onion, optional
Ketchup, optional
Mustard, optional
Nonfat ranch salad dressing,
    optional

Preheat the broiler. Line a baking sheet with foil and spray with cooking spray. Combine the ground turkey, oatmeal, onion powder, pepper flakes, carrots, zucchini, barbecue sauce, ketchup, and garlic in a medium bowl; mix until the ingredients are blended. Shape into six half-inch patties; arrange in a single layer on the baking sheet. Cook for 7 to 8 minutes per side; top with sliced cheese and broil for 45 to 60 seconds, until the cheese is melted. Serve on whole-wheat buns with garnishes as desired.

Nutrition per serving: Calories 292 · Fat 4g · Carbohydrates 35g · Protein 28g · Cholesterol 30mg · Dietary fiber 2g · Sodium 712mg
Exchanges: 3 very lean meat · 2 starch · 1 vegetable
Carb Choices: 2

Be food label savvy! Selecting 99 percent fat-free ground turkey breast over that labeled 85 percent fat-free will save you 130 calories, 15 grams of fat, 5 grams of saturated fat, and 45 grams of cholesterol per 4-ounce serving.

Vegetable-Beef Skillet Meal

EASY   *Serves: 6*

¾ pound extra-lean ground beef   1 cup frozen peas
1 cup diced onion   ¾ cup frozen diced carrots
1 cup diced celery   1 cup uncooked rice
1 cup diced bell pepper   ¾ cup nonfat beef broth
28-ounce can diced tomatoes, do   ¾ cup water
    not drain

Spray a large nonstick skillet with cooking spray; add the ground beef, onion, celery, and bell pepper. Cook, stirring frequently, until the meat is completely browned and the vegetables are tender. Drain any fat from the skillet. Add the tomatoes, peas, carrots, rice, beef broth, and water; bring to a boil over medium-high heat. Reduce heat to low, cover, and cook for 30 to 35 minutes, until the rice is tender.

Nutrition per serving: Calories 247 • Fat 2.7g • Carbohydrates 36g • Protein 16g •
   Cholesterol 30mg • Dietary fiber 4g • Sodium 338mg
Exchanges: 1 lean meat • 2 vegetable • 2 starch
Carb Choices: 2

Unlike some other canned foods, canned tomatoes retain most of their nutrients. In fact, cooked or canned tomatoes contain more lycopene than raw tomatoes. If buying canned tomatoes, choose varieties without added sodium.

Vegetarian Chili with Beans

EASY ▪ DO AHEAD ▪ FREEZE   *Serves: 4*

1¾ cup plus 2 tablespoons canned
   nonfat vegetable broth
2 cups chopped onion
2 cups chopped green bell pepper
1 teaspoon garlic powder
2 tablespoons plus 1 teaspoon
   chili powder
2 teaspoons unsweetened cocoa
   powder
14½-ounce can diced tomatoes,
   lightly drained

1 cup water
1 cup canned chili beans, drained
1 cup canned black beans, drained
1 cup canned garbanzo beans,
   drained
1 cup canned corn kernels, drained
⅛ teaspoon cayenne
Chopped onions, optional
Shredded nonfat cheese, optional
Nonfat sour cream, optional

Spray a large nonstick skillet with cooking spray; add 2 tablespoons of the beef broth to the skillet and heat over medium-high heat. Add the onion, bell pepper, and garlic powder to the skillet; cook, stirring frequently, until the vegetables are softened. Add the chili powder and cocoa powder; cook, stirring constantly, 1 minute to blend. Add the remaining broth, tomatoes, and water; bring to a boil over high heat. Reduce heat to low, cover, and simmer for 15 to 20 minutes. Uncover and stir in the beans, corn, and cayenne; cook over medium heat for 5 to 10 minutes, until completely heated through. Serve with optional garnishes, if desired.

Nutrition per serving: Calories 308 · Fat 2.8g · Carbohydrates 59g · Protein 15g ·
  Cholesterol 0mg · Dietary fiber 9g · Sodium 1,380mg
Exchanges: 3 vegetable · 3 starch
Carb Choices: 4

Like most beans, garbanzo beans are rich in the best sort of fiber—soluble fiber—which helps to eliminate cholesterol from the body. They are a useful source of folate, vitamin E, potassium, iron, manganese, copper, zinc, and calcium. As a high-potassium, low-sodium food they help reduce blood pressure.

Vegetable Lasagna

AVERAGE · DO AHEAD · FREEZE   *Serves: 6*

¾ cup nonfat shredded
   mozzarella cheese, divided
¼ cup nonfat Parmesan cheese,
   divided
1½ cups nonfat cottage cheese
2½ cups low-sodium tomato
   sauce
1 tablespoon plus 1 teaspoon
   Italian seasoning

1 teaspoon onion powder
½ teaspoon garlic powder
⅛ teaspoon pepper
8 ounces lasagna noodles,
   cooked and drained
¾ cup sliced zucchini
¾ cup sliced yellow squash

Preheat the oven to 350 degrees. Spray a 9x13-inch baking dish with cooking spray. Combine 2 tablespoons of mozzarella and 1 tablespoon of Parmesan cheese in a small bowl; mix and set aside. Combine the remaining mozzarella, Parmesan, and cottage cheese in a medium bowl and mix well. Combine the tomato sauce, Italian seasoning, onion powder, garlic powder, and pepper in a medium bowl; mix well. Spread a thin layer of tomato sauce in the bottom of the baking dish; top with a third of the noodles and spread with half the cheese mixture. Top with a layer of zucchini and squash; repeat layering (sauce, noodles, cheese mixture, zucchini, squash, sauce, noodles, sauce). Top with the reserved mozzarella-Parmesan cheese mixture. Cover with heavy-duty foil and bake for 30 to 40 minutes. Remove the foil and bake for 5 to 10 minutes. Remove the baking dish from the oven and let stand for 10 to 15 minutes before serving.

Nutrition per serving: Calories 236 · Fat 1.7g · Carbohydrates 39g · Protein 15g ·
   Cholesterol 37mg · Dietary fiber 2g · Sodium 214mg
Exchanges: 1 very lean meat · 2 starch · 2 vegetable
Carb Choices: 3

Zucchini is a low-calorie, low-fat source of potassium, vitamin A, and a good source of fiber, with 4 grams per cup. Be sure to include the peel to get all the fiber.

Side Dishes

Apricot-Raisin Noodle Kugel

EASY • DO AHEAD • FREEZE   *Serves: 8*

12-ounce package yolk-free egg
   noodles, cooked and drained
1 cup chopped dried apricots
⅔ cup raisins
boiling water
½ cup egg substitute

4 egg whites, lightly beaten
1 cup nonfat half-and-half
½ cup skim milk
½ cup sugar
1 teaspoon cinnamon
⅛ teaspoon nutmeg

Preheat the oven to 350 degrees. Spray a 9x13-inch baking dish with cooking spray. Place the apricots and raisins in a small bowl and cover with boiling water for 5 minutes; drain well. Combine the egg substitute, egg whites, half-and-half, milk, sugar, cinnamon, and nutmeg and mix well; add the cooked noodles and drained apricots and raisins. Toss carefully to mix. Spoon the noodle mixture into the baking dish; cook for 40 to 45 minutes, until set. Remove from the oven and let stand for 5 to 10 minutes before cutting into squares.

Nutrition per serving: Calories 318 • Fat 0.5g • Carbohydrates 68g • Protein 11g •
   Cholesterol <1g • Dietar fiber 4g • Sodium 84mg
Exchanges: ½ very lean meat • 2 starch • 1 fruit • 1 other carb
Carb Choices: 5

Low-fat dairy products can be among the best weight-loss staples, according to researchers at Purdue University who studied a group of women for two years. Those who met the recommended dietary intake (RDI) for calcium (1,000 mg) and ate less than 1,900 calories a day lost an average of six pounds, while women who consumed the same amount of calories but less calcium actually ended up gaining weight. Calcium may help promote the breakdown of the body's fat stores.

Balsamic Glazed Portobello Mushrooms

EASY • DO AHEAD   *Serves: 4*

4 large portobello mushrooms, stems removed	**2 tablespoons brown sugar**
1 cup balsamic vinegar	**1 teaspoon rosemary**
	½ teaspoon garlic powder

Preheat the oven to 450 degrees. Line a baking sheet with foil and spray with cooking spray. Wipe the mushrooms clean with a paper towel (do not wash with water). Place the mushrooms cap side down on the baking sheet. Combine the remaining ingredients and mix well; drizzle the mixture evenly over the mushrooms. Let the mushrooms stand at room temperature for 10 to 15 minutes. Bake for 10 to 15 minutes, until cooked through.

Nutrition per serving: Calories 92 • Fat 0g • Carbohydrates 22g • Protein 1g • Cholesterol 0mg • Dietary fiber 1g • Sodium 14mg

Exchanges: 1 vegetable • 1 other carb

Carb Choices: 1

> Balsamic vinegar has a very strong smell and is high in acidity; therefore, it's best to add it to meals that need a citric taste or for cooking.

Chunky Cinnamon Applesauce

EASY • DO AHEAD   *Serves: 4*

1¾ pounds apples, cored, peeled, and sliced
½ cup sugar
¾ teaspoon cinnamon
½ cup water

Combine the apples, sugar, cinnamon, and water in a large saucepan; bring to a boil over medium-high heat. Reduce the heat to low; simmer, stirring occasionally, until the apples are soft (about 8 to 10 minutes). Remove 1 cup of apples and set aside. Combine the remaining ingredients in a food processor or blender and process until smooth. Pour into a large bowl; add the reserved apples and toss lightly. Cover and refrigerate several hours or overnight before serving.

Nutrition per serving: Calories 208 • Fat 0.7g • Carbohydrates 55g • Protein <1g • Cholesterol 0mg • Dietary fiber 4g • Sodium 1.7mg
Exchanges: 3 fruit • 1 other carb
Carb Choices: 4

Reduce stress with cinnamon. Cinnamon contains a volatile oil that has sedative qualities to help you relax.

Couscous-Veggie Bowl

EASY   *Serves: 6*

2 tablespoons nonfat vegetable
  or chicken broth
¾ cup diced onion
1 medium zucchini, sliced
½ pound eggplant, cubed

15½-ounce can Italian-style
  stewed tomatoes, do not drain
15-ounce can cannellini beans,
  drained
10-ounce package couscous

Spray a large saucepan with cooking spray; add the broth and heat over medium-high heat. Add the onions and cook, stirring frequently, for 5 to 6 minutes, until softened. Add the zucchini and eggplant; cook for 5 to 7 minutes, until soft. Add the stewed tomatoes and beans; bring to a boil over medium-high heat. Reduce heat to low and simmer for 10 to 15 minutes. Cook the couscous according to the package directions. Spoon the vegetables over the cooked couscous; toss lightly and serve.

Nutrition per serving: Calories 271 • Fat 0.7g • Carbohydrates 56g • Protein 11g • Cholesterol 0mg • Dietary fiber 9g • Sodium 504mg

Exchanges: 2 vegetable • 3 starch

Carb Choices: 4

> Eggplant, related to the potato and tomato, is considered a fruit that we consume as vegetable, but botanically it's actually a berry.

Curried Vegetables

EASY   *Serves: 6*

1½ tablespoons nonfat vegetable   4 cups cauliflower florets
  or chicken broth   2¾ cups diced potatoes
1 cup diced onion   15½-ounce can garbanzo beans,
1 tablespoon curry powder   drained
1 teaspoon ground cumin   15-ounce can diced tomatoes
¼ teaspoon cayenne   with garlic and onion
2 teaspoons minced garlic   1½ cups cold water

Spray a large saucepan with cooking spray; add the broth to the pan and heat over medium-high heat. Add the diced onion, curry powder, cumin, and cayenne; cook, stirring frequently, until the onion is lightly browned. Add the minced garlic, cauliflower, potatoes, garbanzo beans, tomatoes, and water to the pan; cover and cook over low heat, stirring occasionally, for 30 to 40 minutes, until the vegetables are tender.

Nutrition per serving: Calories 249 · Fat 2.2g · Carbohydrates 48g · Protein 11g ·
  Cholesterol 0mg · Dietary fiber 5g · Sodium 139mg
Exchanges: 1 vegetable · 3 starch
Carb Choices: 3

Curry powder is a readily available blend of spices that typically contains turmeric, coriander, chiles, cumin, mustard, ginger, fenugreek, garlic, cloves, salt, and any number of other spices.

Fajita-Topped Potatoes

EASY   *Serves: 4*

4 large potatoes
3 tablespoons nonfat chicken or
  vegetable broth
1 cup sliced mushrooms
1 cup diced onion

1 cup chopped green pepper
2 tablespoons diced green chiles,
  drained well
Salsa, optional

Wash the potatoes; dry and poke several times with a fork. Microwave on high for 8 to 9 minutes per potato. Place the potatoes in a 400-degree oven for 15 minutes. Spray a large nonstick skillet with cooking spray. Add the broth to the skillet and heat over medium-high heat. Add the mushrooms, onions, peppers, and chiles to the skillet; cook, stirring frequently, until the vegetables are softened. Remove the potatoes from the oven. Cut the potatoes lengthwise into four slices and arrange on a plate. Top the potatoes with the vegetable mixture and serve with salsa, if desired.

Nutrition per serving: Calories 246 · Fat 0.4g · Carbohydrates 57g · Protein 6g · Cholesterol 0mg · Dietary fiber 7g · Sodium 101mg

Exchanges: 2 starch · 4 vegetable

Carb Choices: 4

Do not leave baked, foil-wrapped potatoes out at room temperature. According to a report in the *Journal of Infectious Diseases,* foil-wrapped potatoes are the perfect breeding ground for bacteria that causes botulism, a form of food poisoning that can lead to muscle paralysis and nerve damage. Remove the foil wrap immediately after baking and refrigerate or eat as soon as possible.

Mango Chutney Rice

EASY   *Serves: 4*

1 cup nonfat vegetable broth   **1 cup dried currants**
1 cup water   **1 teaspoon grated orange peel**
1 cup white rice   **¼ cup mango chutney**

Combine the vegetable broth and water in a large saucepan; bring to a boil over high heat. Add the rice and currants; reduce heat to low, cover and simmer for 20 minutes, until the liquid is absorbed and the rice is tender. Remove the pan from the heat and let stand for 5 minutes. Add the orange peel and chutney to the rice; toss lightly and serve.

Nutrition per serving: Calories 317 • Fat 0.4g • Carbohydrates 74g • Protein 5g • Cholesterol 0mg • Dietary fiber 1g • Sodium 204mg
Exchanges: 1 starch • 4 fruit
Carb Choices: 5

Mangoes are not only rich in vitamins, minerals, antioxidants, and fiber, but are low in calories and sodium. Mangoes are also a good source of vitamins A, B, and C, as well as potassium, calcium, and iron.

Mediterranean Eggplant Pasta

AVERAGE   *Serves: 3 (as main dish), 6 (as side dish)*

28-ounce can diced tomatoes,
  drained
½ teaspoon garlic powder
⅛ teaspoon red pepper flakes
¾ pound eggplant, cut into
  cubes
15-ounce can cannellini beans,
  drained
1 tablespoon dried basil

½ teaspoon dried thyme
2 teaspoons dried parsley
1 teaspoon dried cilantro
12-ounce package penne, rotini,
  rigatoni, or ziti pasta
¼ to ½ cup nonfat chicken or
  vegetable broth, as needed
⅓ cup nonfat Parmesan cheese,
  optional

Spray a large saucepan with cooking spray. Add the tomatoes, garlic powder, and red pepper flakes; cook over medium heat for 5 minutes; reduce the heat to low, cover, and simmer for 5 to 8 minutes. Spray a large nonstick skillet with cooking spray and heat over medium heat. Add the cubed eggplant; cook, stirring frequently, until the eggplant is lightly browned, about 5 to 6 minutes. Add the eggplant to the tomato sauce and cook over medium-low heat until the sauce begins to simmer; reduce heat to low, cover, and simmer for 8 to 10 minutes, until the eggplant is tender. Add the beans, basil, thyme, parsley, and cilantro; cook over medium-low heat for 10 to 15 minutes. While the sauce is simmering, cook the pasta according to package directions; drain well and add to the eggplant sauce. Add broth as needed to moisten. Serve the eggplant pasta with Parmesan cheese, if desired.

Nutrition per serving: Calories 309 • Fat 1.6g • Carbohydrates 62g • Protein 12g •
  Cholesterol 0mg • Dietary fiber 1g • Sodium 560mg
Exchanges: 3 vegetable • 3 starch
Carb Choices: 4

When choosing fruits and vegetables, the more vibrant the color the better. The pigments in the produce contain the majority of healthy antioxidants, which contribute to reduced risk of disease.

Orange Sweet Potatoes

EASY • DO AHEAD *Serves: 4*

1½ pounds sweet potatoes, cut
into 1-inch cubes
½ teaspoon cinnamon
3 tablespoons evaporated
skim milk

1 to 1½ tablespoons orange
marmalade
1 tablespoon orange zest

Spray a square glass baking dish with cooking spray. Arrange the sweet potato cubes in the dish; sprinkle with cinnamon. Microwave on high for 10 to 12 minutes, until soft and cooked through. Mash the potatoes; add the remaining ingredients and mash until smooth and creamy.

Nutrition per serving: Calories 205 • Fat 0.2g • Carbohydrates 49g • Protein 4g • Cholesterol <1mg • Dietary fiber 5g • Sodium 31mg
Exchanges: 2 starch • 1 other carb
Carb Choices: 3

Sweet potatoes, not related to ordinary potatoes, are low in fat yet rich in vitamin E, antioxidants, minerals, iron, beta-carotene, potassium, and zinc.

Orzo Pilaf with Artichokes

EASY   *Serves: 6*

1¾ cups plus 2 tablespoons   1 cup water
   nonfat chicken broth   13¾-ounce can artichoke hearts,
¼ cup chopped green onions   halved and drained well
1 cup uncooked orzo   3 tablespoons nonfat Parmesan
1½ teaspoons Italian seasoning   cheese

Spray a large nonstick skillet with cooking spray; add 2 tablespoons of the chicken broth and heat over medium-high heat. Add the green onions and orzo; cook, stirring constantly, over high heat for 3 to 4 minutes. Add the remaining 1¾ cups of broth, Italian seasoning, and 1 cup water. Bring to a boil over high heat. Reduce heat to low and simmer, uncovered, for 15 to 20 minutes, until all the liquid has been absorbed. Stir in the drained artichoke hearts and Parmesan cheese; toss and serve.

Nutrition per serving: Calories 111 • Fat 0.7g • Carbohydrates 22g • Protein 6g •
   Cholesterol 0mg • Dietary fiber 0g • Sodium 330mg
Exchanges: 1 starch • 1 vegetable
Carb Choices: 1

> People have been using artichokes for their medicinal benefits for hundreds of years. Artichokes contribute to maintaining general health by lowering blood cholesterol and blood sugar, as well as acting as a natural diuretic.

Parmesan Pasta Pilaf

EASY   *Serves: 6*

1¼ cups plus 2 tablespoons
    nonfat chicken or vegetable
    broth
½ cup uncooked vermicelli or
    spaghettini, broken into small
    pieces
2 teaspoons instant minced
    onion

1 cup long-grain white rice,
    uncooked
1¼ cups hot water
¼ teaspoon crushed bay leaf
3 tablespoons nonfat Parmesan
    cheese

Spray a large nonstick skillet with cooking spray; add 2 tablespoons of the broth and heat over medium-high heat. Add the vermicelli and onion to the skillet; cook over medium-high heat, stirring frequently, until the vermicelli is lightly browned. Add the rice, remaining 1¼ cups of broth, water, and bay leaf. Reduce heat to low, cover, and simmer for 15 to 20 minutes, until the liquid is absorbed. Remove from heat; fluff with a fork and let stand for 5 to 10 minutes before serving. Just before serving, sprinkle with Parmesan cheese.

Nutrition per serving: Calories 158 • Fat 0.4g • Carbohydrates 33g • Protein 5g •
    Cholesterol 0mg • Dietary fiber <1g • Sodium 204mg
Exchanges: 2 starch
Carb Choices: 2

There are many varieties of rice that differ in nutritional value depending on the type of starch that makes up the grain. Long-grain white rice has the most amylase and the least amylopectin, so it tends to be the fluffiest and least sticky.

Parmesan Vegetable Bake

AVERAGE   *Serves: 6*

15½-ounce can diced tomatoes
    with garlic and onion; do not
    drain
1 small onion, peeled and sliced
1 small green bell pepper, seeded
    and diced
¼ pound fresh asparagus, cut
    into 1-inch pieces
¼ pound fresh okra, cut into
    ½-inch pieces

1 tablespoon lemon juice
¾ teaspoon Italian seasoning
2 small zucchini, cut into 1-inch
    cubes
1 small eggplant, peeled and cut
    into 1-inch cubes
3 tablespoons nonfat Parmesan
    cheese

Preheat the oven to 325 degrees. Spray a 9x13-inch baking dish with cooking spray. In a large bowl, combine the tomatoes with liquid, onion, bell pepper, asparagus, okra, lemon juice, and Italian seasoning. Toss lightly; spoon the mixture into the baking dish. Cover with heavy-duty foil and bake for 15 minutes. Add the zucchini and eggplant; cover and bake for 60 to 70 minutes, until the vegetables are tender. Sprinkle with Parmesan cheese and serve.

Nutrition per serving: Calories 61 • Fat 0.2g • Carbohydrates 12g • Protein 3g •
    Cholesterol 0mg • Dietary fiber 2g • Sodium 142mg
Exchanges: 3 vegetable
Carb Choices: 1

Boosting the amount of blue/purple vegetables and fruits in your diet may lower the risk of some cancers, promote urinary tract health, improve memory function, and promote healthy aging due to phytochemicals such as anthocyanins and phenolics found in blueberries, purple grapes, raisins, and eggplant.

Pasta with Vegetarian Sauce

EASY • DO AHEAD • FREEZE   *Serves: 3 (as main dish), 6 (as side dish)*

2 tablespoons nonfat vegetable
  or chicken broth
2 tablespoons onion powder
¾ teaspoon garlic powder
¾ cup sliced zucchini
¾ cup sliced yellow squash
1½ tablespoons Italian
  seasoning

15½-ounce can diced tomatoes
  with garlic and onion, lightly
  drained
8-ounce can tomato sauce
6-ounce can tomato paste
1 cup water
3 cups cooked spaghetti, angel
  hair pasta, or vermicelli

Spray a large nonstick skillet or Dutch oven with cooking spray; add the broth, onion powder, and garlic powder and heat over medium-high heat. Add the zucchini and squash; cook, stirring frequently, for about 5 minutes, until softened. Add the Italian seasoning, tomatoes, tomato sauce, tomato paste, and water; bring to a boil over high heat. Reduce heat to low, cover, and simmer for 30 to 45 minutes. Serve sauce over cooked pasta.

Nutrition per serving: Calories 158 • Fat 0.8g • Carbohydrates 33g • Protein 6g •
  Cholesterol 0mg • Dietary fiber 4g • Sodium 381mg
Exchanges: 3 vegetable • 1 starch
Carb Choices: 2

Tomato puree or tomato paste concentrates the nutrients found in tomatoes. One ounce of puree contains twice as much vitamin C and 20 percent more beta-carotene than one ounce of fresh tomato. Tomato paste is even more nutritious, containing twice as much beta-carotene.

Potato Quesadillas

AVERAGE • DO AHEAD   *Serves:* 6

6 8-inch low-fat flour tortillas
½ to ¾ cup nonfat chicken or
   vegetable broth, divided and
   used as needed
1 small onion, thinly sliced
16-ounce package pre-cooked
   roasted onion potato cubes
1 tablespoon chopped fresh
   parsley

Pepper to taste
1½ cup nonfat shredded
   cheddar cheese, divided
6 tablespoons canned diced
   green chiles, drained
¾ cup nonfat sour cream,
   optional
¾ to 1 cup chunky-style salsa,
   optional

Preheat the oven to 400 degrees. Line a baking sheet(s) with foil and spray with cooking spray. Arrange 3 tortillas in a single layer on the baking sheet(s). Spray a large nonstick skillet with cooking spray; add 2 tablespoons of the broth and heat over medium-high heat. Add the onions; cook, stirring frequently, until the onions are lightly browned. Add the potatoes and ½ cup of the broth; cook over medium-low heat until all the liquid has been absorbed. Stir in the parsley and season with pepper to taste. Divide the potato mixture among the tortillas, spreading evenly almost to the edges. Sprinkle each tortilla with ¼ cup of shredded cheese and 1 tablespoon green chiles. Top with the remaining tortillas; spray lightly with cooking spray. Bake for 5 to 6 minutes; carefully turn the tortillas over, spray lightly with cooking spray, and bake for 5 to 8 more minutes, until lightly browned and the cheese is melted. Remove from the oven and let stand for 3 minutes before slicing into wedges. If desired, serve with nonfat sour cream and/or salsa.

Nutrition per serving: Calories 246 • Fat 0.5g • Carbohydrates 44g • Protein 14g •
   Cholesterol 0mg • Dietary fiber 4g • Sodium 933mg
Exchanges: 2½ starch • 1 very lean meat • 1 vegetable
Carb Choices: 3

> Parsley has been used throughout the ages as a blood purifier; eating parsley on a regular basis can help your body by lowering the heart rate and blood pressure.

Roasted Vegetables

EASY • DO AHEAD   *Serves: 6*

¼ cup nonfat chicken or
  vegetable broth
1 tablespoon minced garlic
1½ teaspoons dried thyme
  leaves

1½ pounds medium red
  potatoes, quartered
1 pound baby carrots
1 medium Vidalia onion, peeled
  and cut into wedges

Preheat the oven to 350 degrees. Line a baking sheet with foil and spray with cooking spray. Combine the chicken broth, garlic, and thyme in a large bowl; add the vegetables and toss until coated. Spread the vegetables in an even layer on the baking sheet; drizzle with the remaining sauce. Bake for 50 to 55 minutes, until tender. Great side dish with meat loaf, chicken, or fish.

Nutrition per serving: Calories 150 • Fat 0.3g • Carbohydrates 35g • Protein 3g •
  Cholesterol 0mg • Dietary fiber 6g • Sodium 66mg
Exchanges: 1 starch • 3 vegetable
Carb Choices: 2

When purchasing garlic, make sure it is still firm and hasn't sprouted. Store garlic in a cool, dark place and do not refrigerate or freeze.

Sesame Potato Sticks

EASY • DO AHEAD   *Serves: 4*

**4 large baking potatoes, cut
 lengthwise into wedges**
¼ cup low-sodium teriyaki sauce

½ cup Corn Flake crumbs
½ teaspoon garlic powder
2 teaspoons sesame seeds

Preheat the oven to 450 degrees. Line a baking sheet(s) with foil and spray with cooking spray. Arrange the potato wedges on the baking sheet(s) in a single layer. Brush the wedges with the teriyaki sauce. Combine the Corn Flake crumbs, garlic powder, and sesame seeds in a bowl or zip-top bag and mix well. Sprinkle the crumb mixture over the potatoes; bake for 35 to 40 minutes, until lightly browned and cooked through.

Nutrition per serving: Calories 282 • Fat 0.9g • Carbohydrates 62g • Protein 6g •
    Cholesterol 0mg • Dietary fiber 6g • Sodium 452mg
Exchanges: 3 starch • 1 other carb
Carb Choices: 4

> The nutrient value of sesame seeds varies from one seed to another, but they all contain protein, oils, lecithin, minerals, and more. Unhulled seeds contain more calcium than hulled seeds.

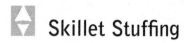 # Skillet Stuffing

EASY ● DO AHEAD   *Serves: 6*

1 cup plus 2 tablespoons nonfat
  vegetable or chicken broth,
  divided
10-ounce package frozen
  seasoning vegetables (onion,
  celery, bell peppers)
6-ounce package cornbread
  stuffing mix

20-ounce can crushed pineapple,
  undrained
6-ounce package stuffing cubes
1 cup dried cranberries
¼ cup sliced water chestnuts

Spray a large nonstick skillet with cooking spray. Add 2 tablespoons of the broth and heat over medium-high heat. Add the seasoning vegetables; cook, stirring frequently, until the vegetables are softened. Stir in the cornbread from stuffing mix, crushed pineapple with juice, and the remaining 1 cup of broth. Bring to a boil over high heat. Remove the skillet from the heat. Add the stuffing cubes and cornbread stuffing mix, cranberries, and water chestnuts. Mix well. Heat, stirring constantly, over low heat until heated through.

Nutrition per serving: Calories 339 • Fat 1.2g • Carbohydrates 76g • Protein 7g •
  Cholesterol 0mg • Dietary fiber 3g • Sodium 871mg
Exchanges: 3 vegetable • 2 starch • 2 fruit
Carb Choices: 5

Red fruits and vegetables such as cranberries, raspberries, red grapes, strawberries, red peppers, red potatoes, red onions, and tomatoes, are known for such phytochemicals as lycopene and anthocyanins, which contribute to heart health, memory function, reduced risk of certain cancers, and urinary-tract health.

Soyfully Rich Couscous

EASY   *Serves: 4*

1 cup water
1 cup frozen shelled edamame,
   thawed and drained
¾ cup uncooked couscous

1 teaspoon dried parsley
2 teaspoons lemon juice
¾ teaspoon grated lemon rind
Pepper to taste

Pour the water into a medium saucepan and bring to a boil over high heat. Add the thawed edamame; cook for 30 to 60 seconds. Stir in the couscous, parsley, lemon juice, lemon rind, and pepper. Remove the saucepan from the heat, cover tightly, and let stand for 5 to 6 minutes. Fluff with a fork before serving.

Nutrition per serving: Calories 169 · Fat 2g · Carbohydrates 30g · Protein 8g ·
   Cholesterol 0mg · Dietary fiber 6g · Sodium 93mg
Exchanges: 2 starch
Carb Choices: 2

Edamame are fresh soybeans picked at the adolescent stage, so they can be eaten when they are still young and tender. These beans have a mild, slightly nutty flavor and are the only beans considered to be a "complete protein," providing the same essential amino acids as animal protein.

Spaghetti Squash with Chunky Tomato Sauce

EASY *Serves: 4*

1½ pound spaghetti squash,
   halved and seeded
1 tablespoon nonfat vegetable or
   chicken broth
1 teaspoon minced garlic
1 tablespoon onion powder
28-ounce can diced tomatoes
   with garlic and onion

3 tablespoons tomato paste
1 teaspoon white wine vinegar
2 teaspoons Italian seasoning
½ teaspoon red pepper flakes
Nonfat Parmesan cheese,
   optional
Fresh basil leaves, chopped fine,
   optional

Preheat the oven to 375 degrees. Line a baking sheet with foil and spray with cooking spray. Place the seeded squash halves, flesh side down, on the baking sheet. Bake for 30 to 35 minutes, until softened. Spray a large nonstick skillet with cooking spray; add the broth and heat over medium-high heat. Add the minced garlic and onion powder; cook over medium heat for 1 to 2 minutes. Add the tomatoes, tomato paste, wine vinegar, Italian seasoning, and pepper flakes to the skillet. Cook over medium heat, stirring frequently, for 25 to 30 minutes; reduce the heat to medium-low if the sauce begins to boil. Remove the squash from the oven and pull the strands from the shell. Place the "spaghetti strands" in a large bowl; pour the sauce over the top and garnish with Parmesan cheese and chopped basil leaves, if desired.

Nutrition per serving: Calories 99 • Fat 0.5g • Carbohydrates 19g • Protein 3g •
   Cholesterol 0mg • Dietary fiber 4g • Sodium 446mg
Exchanges: 4 vegetable
Carb Choices: 1

Spaghetti squash is available in two varieties: standard spaghetti squash has a bright yellow outer shell and a creamy-colored inside, while the "orangetti" variety has orange-colored flesh. Although the varieties differ in inside flesh color, both varieties taste the same. When calculating how much spaghetti squash to purchase for a recipe, know that a four-pound spaghetti squash will produce approximately five cups of usable spaghetti-like flesh.

Spanish Rice

EASY   *Serves: 4*

1 cup plus 2 tablespoons nonfat
   chicken broth
1 cup water
1 cup long-grain rice
1 cup diced onion
1 teaspoon minced garlic
2 cups chopped red and green
   bell pepper

8 ounces sliced mushrooms
16-ounce can crushed tomatoes,
   do not drain
2 teaspoons fresh chopped
   basil
Pepper to taste

Combine 1 cup of the broth and the water in a large saucepan; bring to a boil over high heat. Add the rice; return to a boil. Reduce heat to low, cover, and simmer for 15 to 20 minutes, until the liquid is absorbed and the rice is tender. Spray a large skillet with cooking spray; add the remaining 2 tablespoons of chicken broth and heat over medium-high heat. Add the onions, garlic, bell peppers, and mushrooms; cook, stirring frequently, for 5 to 6 minutes, until the vegetables are softened. Add the tomatoes and basil; cook over medium-high heat, stirring constantly, until the mixture is heated through. Reduce heat to low; add the cooked rice, toss, and serve. Season with pepper as desired.

Nutrition per serving: Calories 239 · Fat 0.8g · Carbohydrates 50g · Protein 7g ·
   Cholesterol 0mg · Dietary fiber 3g · Sodium 405mg
Exchanges: 2 starch · 4 vegetable
Carb Choices: 3

> White fruits and vegetables such as mushrooms, onions, potatoes, jicama, cauliflower, ginger, garlic, and bananas contribute to heart health, maintain healthy cholesterol levels, and reduce the risk of some cancers.

Spinach Bake Au Gratin

EASY · DO AHEAD   *Serves: 6*

**16-ounce package frozen
    chopped spinach, thawed
    and drained**
1 tablespoon onion powder
2 cups nonfat cottage cheese
½ cup egg substitute
2 egg whites, lightly beaten

**¼ cup plus 3 tablespoons nonfat
    Parmesan cheese, divided**
¼ teaspoon dried basil
¼ teaspoon pepper
**1 large tomato, sliced ¼-inch
    thick**
¼ cup Corn Flake crumbs

Preheat the oven to 375 degrees. Spray a shallow baking dish with cooking spray. Combine the spinach, onion powder, cottage cheese, egg substitute, egg whites, ¼ cup of the Parmesan cheese, basil, and pepper in a large bowl; mix until the ingredients are completely blended. Spoon the spinach mixture into the baking dish; arrange the tomato slices on top. Combine the Corn Flake crumbs and the remaining 3 tablespoons of Parmesan cheese in a zip-top bag or bowl and mix well; sprinkle the crumb mixture over the tomatoes. Bake the casserole for 25 to 30 minutes, until bubbly and lightly browned.

Nutrition per serving: Calories 91 · Fat 0.2g · Carbohydrates 12g · Protein 11g ·
    Cholesterol 2mg · Dietary fiber 2g · Sodium 301mg
Exchanges: 2 vegetable · 1 very lean meat
Carb Choices: 1

When selecting tomatoes, be sure to pick those with the most brilliant shades of red, indicating the highest amounts of beta-carotene and lycopene.

Spinach Mashed Potatoes

EASY   *Serves: 4*

1-pound 4-ounce package diced potatoes	10-ounce package frozen chopped spinach, thawed and drained
2 to 3 tablespoons nonfat chicken broth, divided	¼ cup nonfat half-and-half
¾ teaspoon minced garlic	Pepper to taste

Spray a large nonstick skillet with cooking spray; add the diced potatoes and cover with water. Cover the pan and cook over low heat until the potatoes are softened. Drain well and place in a medium bowl. Mash the potatoes until smooth. Spray the skillet again with cooking spray; add 1 tablespoon of the chicken broth and heat over medium-high heat. Add the garlic and spinach; cook, stirring frequently, until the spinach is wilted. Add the spinach to the mashed potatoes; stir in the half-and-half, 1 to 2 tablespoons of chicken broth, and pepper to taste. Serve immediately.

Nutrition per serving: Calories 161 • Fat 0.1g • Carbohydrates 35g • Protein 6g • Cholesterol 0mg • Dietary fiber 5g • Sodium 217mg

Exchanges: 1 starch • 2 vegetable • ½ other carb

Carb Choices: 2

> Eating crushed garlic on a regular basis can contribute to lower blood pressure, reduced risk of stroke, increased immunity, and better circulation.

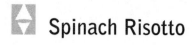

Spinach Risotto

AVERAGE

Serves: 4

4 cups plus 1½ tablespoons
  nonfat chicken or vegetable
  broth
¾ cup diced onion
1½ teaspoons minced garlic
1 cup Arborio rice
10-ounce package frozen
  chopped spinach, thawed and
  drained

¼ teaspoon dried Italian
  seasoning
¼ cup nonfat Parmesan cheese
1 teaspoon rice vinegar
Pepper to taste

Pour 4 cups of the broth into a microwave-safe bowl; bring to a boil on high heat. Cover and set aside to keep warm. Spray a 3-quart saucepan with cooking spray; add the remaining 1½ tablespoons of broth and heat over medium-high heat. Add the onion and garlic; cook, stirring frequently, about 5 minutes, until the onion and garlic are softened. Add the rice and mix well. Add 1 cup of the warm broth; cook, stirring constantly, until the liquid is absorbed, about 5 minutes. Repeat the procedure with the remaining 3 cups of warm broth, until most of the liquid has been absorbed. Add the spinach and Italian seasoning; cook, stirring constantly, until all the liquid is absorbed. Stir in the Parmesan cheese and rice vinegar. Season with pepper as desired and serve immediately.

Nutrition per serving: Calories 233 • Fat 1g • Carbohydrates 46g • Protein 11g •
  Cholesterol 0mg • Dietary fiber 3g • Sodium 909mg
Exchanges: 2 starch • 1 vegetable • ½ other carb
Carb Choices: 3

Eat up! Two cups of steamed greens (spinach, kale, collards, and mustard greens) contain less than 100 calories and 1 gram of fat while providing substantial protective nutrients that fight a variety of diseases.

Steamed Asparagus and Peas with Brown Rice

EASY

Serves: 6

⅔ cup water
¾ cup nonfat vegetable or
  chicken broth
½ teaspoon onion powder
1½ pounds fresh asparagus
  spears, trimmed and cut into
  1-inch pieces

10-ounce package frozen
  baby peas
3 tablespoons chopped
  pimientos, drained
3 cups cooked brown rice

Spray a large nonstick skillet with cooking spray; add the water, broth, and onion powder. Bring to a boil over high heat. Add the asparagus and peas; reduce heat to medium-low, cover, and simmer for 5 minutes. Uncover the skillet; add the pimientos and cook until most of the liquid has been absorbed. Serve the vegetables over ½ cup of brown rice per serving.

Nutrition per serving: Calories 180 • Fat 1.4g • Carbohydrates 35g • Protein 8g •
  Cholesterol 0mg • Dietary fiber 1g • Sodium 107mg
Exchanges: 1 vegetable • 2 starch
Carb Choices: 2

Keep asparagus fresh by cutting off one inch from the bottom of the stems and standing the stalks in a container tall enough to hold them upright. Add about two inches of water, cover loosely with a plastic bag, and refrigerate. Add more water as needed to keep the bottoms covered.

Stir-Fry Chinese Vegetables

EASY   *Serves: 4*

1 tablespoon nonfat chicken or
   vegetable broth
1 cup chopped onion
1 cup shredded carrots
10-ounce package frozen snow
   peas, thawed and drained
¼ cup diced celery

¼ pound bean sprouts
2 tablespoons low-sodium soy
   sauce
2 teaspoons lemon juice
½ teaspoon sugar
Pepper to taste

Spray a large nonstick skillet with cooking spray; add the broth and heat over medium-high heat. Add the onions, carrots, snow peas, and celery to the skillet; cook, stirring constantly for 3 to 4 minutes, until the vegetables are tender crisp. Add the bean sprouts and cook for 1 minute. Combine the soy sauce, lemon juice, and sugar in a small bowl; mix well. Pour the sauce over the vegetables and cook, stirring constantly, for 1 to 2 minutes, until coated and heated through. Vegetables can be served alone or over rice, pasta, or baked potato.

Nutrition per serving: Calories 70 • Fat 0.3g • Carbohydrates 14g • Protein 4g •
   Cholesterol 0mg • Dietary fiber 2g • Sodium 345mg
Exchanges: 3 vegetable
Carb Choices: 1

Snow peas, like all peas, are a type of legume.

Vegetable Couscous

EASY • DO AHEAD   *Serves: 4*

2½ cups plus 1 tablespoon   1½ cups asparagus, cut into
   nonfat chicken or vegetable   1-inch pieces
   broth, divided   1¼ cups sliced bell peppers
1 cup diced onion   1½ cups diced cucumber
1 teaspoon minced garlic   1 cup uncooked couscous
½ teaspoon mustard powder   ½ cup petite-cut diced
½ teaspoon ground cumin   tomatoes with roasted garlic
½ teaspoon ground ginger   and sweet onions, drained
1 cup baby carrots, cut in half   ¼ cup minced fresh parsley

Spray a large nonstick skillet with cooking spray; add 1 tablespoon of the broth and heat over medium-high heat. Add the onion and garlic to the skillet; cook, stirring frequently, for about 5 minutes, until tender. Add the mustard powder, cumin, and ginger; cook, stirring constantly, for about 1 minute. Add the remaining 2½ cups of broth to the skillet; bring to a boil over high heat. Add the carrots, asparagus, and bell peppers; reduce heat to medium-low, cover, and cook for 5 to 6 minutes. Add the cucumber; cook for 2 to 3 minutes. Increase the heat to medium-high; bring to a boil (uncovered). Immediately stir in the couscous; cover the skillet, remove from heat, and let stand for 5 minutes. Add the diced tomatoes and parsley; toss and fluff with a fork.

Nutrition per serving: Calories 251 • Fat 1.1g • Carbohydrates 49g • Protein 11g •
   Cholesterol 0mg • Dietary fiber 11g • Sodium 590mg
Exchanges: 2½ starch • 2 vegetable
Carb Choices: 3

> Onions, garlic, chili peppers, ginger, pineapple, and tea discourage blood clotting. Onions, garlic, and chili peppers can also help blood flow more freely by dilating the blood vessels.

Vegetarian Stuffed Peppers

AVERAGE • DO AHEAD • FREEZE   *Serves: 4*

4 large bell peppers, cut in half
   lengthwise, stems removed,
   and seeded
1½ cups nonfat vegetable broth
½ cup canned corn kernels
¾ cup diced onion
¾ cup diced carrots
½ teaspoon dried thyme

½ teaspoon minced garlic
1¼ cups instant brown rice,
   uncooked
1 cup nonfat shredded
   mozzarella cheese
4 tablespoons nonfat Parmesan
   cheese

Preheat the oven to 400 degrees. Spray a 9x13-inch baking dish with cooking spray. Place the bell peppers in a single layer in a baking dish; cover with plastic wrap and microwave on high for 2 to 3 minutes until tender. Spray a medium saucepan with cooking spray; add the broth, corn, onions, carrots, thyme, and garlic. Bring to a boil over medium-high heat. Stir in the rice; reduce the heat to low, cover, and simmer for 8 to 10 minutes, until the liquid is absorbed. Remove from the heat and fluff the rice with a fork. Add the mozzarella and Parmesan cheeses to the rice. Spoon the mixture into the pepper shells; cover the dish with foil and bake for 15 to 20 minutes, until the cheese is melted and the vegetables are tender.

Nutrition per serving: Calories 209 • Fat 1.2g • Carbohydrates 34g • Protein 16g •
   Cholesterol 0mg • Dietary fiber 5g • Sodium 632mg
Exchanges: 1 vegetable • 2 starch • 1 very lean meat
Carb Choices: 2

Green and yellow-orange foods are rich in vitamins; they also contain potent carotenoids and other phytochemicals that slow damage to cells, protect against cancer and heart disease, boost the immune system, and generally defend our bodies against illness.

Desserts

 ## Angel Food Cake with Honey-Yogurt Fruit

EASY • DO AHEAD   *Serves: 4*

½ cup nonfat vanilla yogurt
2 tablespoons honey
1 cup fresh pineapple chunks
2 bananas, cut into 1-inch slices

1 cup seedless grapes
8-ounce can mandarin oranges,
  drained well
4 slices prepared angel food cake

Combine the yogurt and honey in a small bowl and mix well. Combine the pineapple, bananas, grapes, and oranges in a medium bowl; pour the yogurt mixture over the top and toss lightly. Cover and refrigerate for 15 to 20 minutes. Arrange one angel food cake slice on each plate and top with the honey-yogurt fruit mixture.

Nutrition per serving: Calories 309 • Fat 0.6g • Carbohydrates 73g • Protein 6g •
   Cholesterol 1mg • Dietary fiber 2g • Sodium 166mg
Exchanges: 5 other carb
Carb Choices: 5

University of Illinois food scientists have discovered that honey is rich in heart-protecting antioxidants. In studies, honey slowed the oxidation of bad LDL cholesterol in human blood.

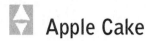 # Apple Cake

EASY · DO AHEAD · FREEZE   *Serves: 16*

¼ cup nonfat vanilla yogurt
¼ cup applesauce
¼ cup egg substitute
2 egg whites
1 teaspoon vanilla
¾ cup sugar
¾ cup brown sugar
1¾ cups all-purpose flour

1 cup whole-wheat flour
½ cup wheat germ
1½ teaspoons cinnamon
½ teaspoon nutmeg
2 cups peeled and chopped
   apples
Cinnamon-sugar topping,
   optional

Preheat the oven to 350 degrees. Spray a 9x13-inch baking dish with cooking spray. Combine the yogurt, applesauce, egg substitute, egg whites, vanilla, sugar, and brown sugar in a large bowl; mix until blended smooth. Combine the all-purpose flour, whole-wheat flour, wheat germ, cinnamon, and nutmeg in a zip-top bag; shake until the ingredients are well mixed. Add the dry ingredients to the mixing bowl, blending until the ingredients are moistened. Fold in the apples and mix lightly. Spread the batter in the baking dish. Bake for 40 to 45 minutes, until a toothpick inserted in the center comes out clean. Cool completely. Just before serving, sprinkle with cinnamon-sugar, if desired.

Nutrition per serving: Calories 182 · Fat 0.7g · Carbohydrates 41g · Protein 4g ·
   Cholesterol 0mg · Dietary fiber 2g · Sodium 25mg
Exchanges: 2½ other carb
Carb Choices: 3

When the University of Minnesota researchers studied eating and activity patterns of 285 teens for three years, they uncovered a secret weapon against obesity, diabetes, and heart disease: whole grains. Whole grains help you feel full longer, which may prevent overeating; improve how well your body metabolizes sugar; and provide protective compounds that get stripped away when the grain is processed.

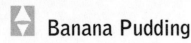 # Banana Pudding

EASY • DO AHEAD   *Serves: 4*

2 bananas, divided

1 teaspoon lemon juice

2 tablespoons nonfat half-
and-half

1 tablespoon plus 1 teaspoon
sugar

1 teaspoon vanilla

1 cup nonfat vanilla yogurt

1 teaspoon cinnamon-sugar
mixture

Peel and slice 1 banana; reserve the other banana until ready to serve. Combine the sliced banana, 1 teaspoon lemon juice, half-and-half, sugar, and vanilla in a food processor or blender; process until smooth and creamy. Pour the banana mixture into a bowl; fold in the yogurt. Cover and refrigerate for at least 6 hours or overnight. Divide the pudding among four dessert dishes. Slice the remaining banana and garnish the pudding. Sprinkle each with ¼ teaspoon cinnamon-sugar.

Nutrition per serving: Calories 102 • Fat 0.2g • Carbohydrates 23g • Protein 3g •
   Cholesterol 1mg • Dietary fiber 1g • Sodium 36mg
Exchanges: 1½ other carb
Carb Choices: 2

Bananas develop their best eating quality after they are harvested. Sensitive to cool temperatures, bananas should never be refrigerated.

Chocolate Almond Angel Food Cake with Strawberry Slices

AVERAGE ◦ DO AHEAD ◦ FREEZE   *Serves: 10*

12 egg whites

1¼ cups sugar, divided

1 teaspoon cream of tartar

1 teaspoon almond extract

½ teaspoon vanilla extract

¾ cup cake flour

¼ cup unsweetened cocoa powder

2 cups sliced strawberries

2 tablespoons nonfat Cool Whip
    per serving or 1 tablespoon
    nonfat chocolate syrup, optional

Preheat the oven to 350 degrees. Lightly spray a 10-inch tube pan with cooking spray. Place the egg whites in a large bowl; add ¼ cup of the sugar and whip with an electric mixer until frothy. Add the cream of tartar. Whip the egg whites until stiff. Carefully fold in the remaining cup of sugar a little at a time. Fold in the almond and vanilla extracts, mixing very lightly. Combine the cake flour and cocoa powder in a zip-top bag; shake vigorously until the ingredients are completely mixed. Gradually add the flour mixture to the egg mixture, mixing carefully after each addition. Pour the batter into the tube pan; bake for 40 to 45 minutes, until a toothpick inserted in the center comes out clean. Let the cake sit for 5 minutes; invert the pan onto a plate or wire rack and cool completely. Serve with sliced strawberries, nonfat Cool Whip, and/or chocolate syrup as desired.

Nutrition per serving: Calories 157 • Fat 0.4g • Carbohydrates 35g • Protein 6g •
    Cholesterol 0mg • Dietary fiber 1g • Sodium 68mg

Exchanges: 2 other carb

Carb Choices: 2

According to a study at the University of California at Davis, consuming just a handful of semisweet chocolate chips may contain enough disease-fighting compounds to help ward off cardiovascular disease and stroke. Consuming four times that amount produced the same effect, so there's no need to go chocolate crazy.

Cinnamon Pears with Oat Crunch Topping

EASY • DO AHEAD   *Serves: 6*

**6 cups peeled and thinly sliced
    pears**
¼ cup water
½ cup brown sugar, divided
2 tablespoons all-purpose flour
**1½ teaspoons ground cinnamon,
    divided**

1 cup quick-cooking oatmeal
¼ cup toasted wheat germ
**3 tablespoons nonfat vanilla
    yogurt**
**Nonfat frozen yogurt (½ cup per
    serving), optional**

Preheat the oven to 350 degrees. Spray an 8-inch baking dish with cooking spray. Combine the pears and water in a large bowl; add ¼ cup of the brown sugar, the flour, and ¾ teaspoon of the cinnamon; mix until the pears are coated. Spoon the pear mixture into the baking dish. Combine the oatmeal, wheat germ, the remaining ¼ cup brown sugar, and the remaining ¾ teaspoon of cinnamon in a medium bowl; mix well. Gradually add the yogurt, mixing with your fingertips until the ingredients are moistened and crumbly. Add just enough yogurt to make a crumb mixture. Sprinkle the crumbs over the pears and bake for 30 to 35 minutes, until bubbly hot and lightly browned on top. Serve with nonfat frozen yogurt, if desired.

Nutrition per serving: Calories 249 • Fat 2g • Carbohydrates 57g • Protein 4g •
    Cholesterol <1mg • Dietary fiber 6g • Sodium 11mg
Exchanges: 4 other carb
Carb Choices: 4

Wheat germ is the nutrient-packed center of the wheatberry; it is the source of all vitamins, minerals, and proteins, providing a nutty flavor to cereals and baked goods. Wheat germ, along with sunflower products, almonds, and sweet potatoes, is rich in vitamin E, the antioxidant most strongly linked with a lower risk of angina and heart attack.

Cinnamon Raisin Peach Crisp

EASY • DO AHEAD   *Serves: 8*

½ cup quick-cooking oats,
   uncooked
1 tablespoon all-purpose flour
1½ tablespoons brown sugar
1 teaspoon cinnamon, divided
1¼ tablespoons nonfat vanilla
   yogurt

3 pounds fresh peaches, peeled
   and sliced
½ cup raisins
⅛ teaspoon ground nutmeg

Preheat the oven to 350 degrees. Spray a 2-quart shallow baking dish with cooking spray. Combine the oatmeal, flour, brown sugar, and ½ teaspoon of the cinnamon in a small bowl and mix well; add the yogurt and mix with your fingertips until moistened and crumbly. Combine the peaches, raisins, the remaining ½ teaspoon of cinnamon, and nutmeg in a large bowl; mix well. Spoon the peaches into a baking dish; sprinkle the oat mixture over the top. Bake for 35 to 40 minutes, until bubbly and lightly browned on top. Serve with nonfat frozen yogurt, if desired (½ cup per serving).

Nutrition per serving: Calories 135 • Fat 0.5g • Carbohydrates 33g • Protein 2g • Cholesterol 0mg • Dietary fiber 3g • Sodium 3mg
Exchanges: 2 other carb
Carb Choices: 2

Oatmeal has one of the best amino acid profiles of all grains. Amino acids are essential proteins that help facilitate optimum functioning of the body.

Cran-Apricot Oatmeal Bars

EASY • DO AHEAD • FREEZE   *Serves: 12*

1 cup quick-cooking oatmeal
½ cup whole-wheat flour
½ cup all-purpose flour
¾ teaspoon cinnamon
⅔ cup brown sugar

¼ teaspoon baking soda
¼ cup nonfat vanilla yogurt
¼ cup cranberry juice
1¼ cups apricot preserves

Preheat the oven to 325 degrees. Spray an 8x12-inch baking dish with cooking spray. In a medium bowl, combine the oatmeal, whole-wheat flour, all-purpose flour, cinnamon, brown sugar, and baking soda; using your fingertips, mix the ingredients until crumbly. Combine the yogurt and cranberry juice in a small bowl; mix well. Drizzle the mixture over the oats and mix with your fingertips, just until moist and crumbly. Press half the mixture into the bottom of the baking dish. Spread the preserves over the top; sprinkle with the remaining oat mixture. Bake for 30 to 45 minutes, until lightly browned and cooked through. Remove from the oven and cool completely before cutting into squares. These bars can be stored in an airtight container at room temperature or packaged and frozen.

Nutrition per serving: Calories 204 • Fat 0.5g • Carbohydrates 48g • Protein 2g •
Cholesterol <1mg • Dietary fiber 1g • Sodium 28mg
Exchanges: 3 other carb
Carb Choices: 3

Cranberry juice enhances the absorption of vitamin B_{12}, a vitamin that is difficult for some older people with too little stomach acid, or those taking acid suppressors, to absorb.

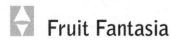

Fruit Fantasia

EASY • DO AHEAD   *Serves: 6*

1 cup sliced peaches
1 papaya, peeled, seeded, and cut
   into large chunks
1 cup pineapple chunks
1⅓ cups strawberries, hulled
   and sliced
2 kiwifruit, peeled and sliced

¾ pound watermelon, peeled,
   seeded, and cut into chunks
1 orange, peeled and cut
⅔ cup sugar
¾ cup nonfat Cool Whip, regular
   or vanilla flavored
Cinnamon

Combine the peaches, papaya, pineapple, strawberries, kiwi, watermelon, and orange in a large bowl. Sprinkle with the sugar and toss to coat. Divide the mixture among 6 dessert dishes and top each with 2 tablespoons of Cool Whip. Sprinkle with a dash of cinnamon and serve.

Nutrition per serving: Calories 183 • Fat 0.6g • Carbohydrates 46g • Protein 1g •
   Cholesterol 0mg • Dietary fiber 3g • Sodium 6mg
Exchanges: 2 fruit • 1 other carb
Carb Choices: 3

Ripe papayas, available year-round, contain papain enzymes, which promote digestion. While the papaya skin is not edible, its seeds are.

Fresh Fruit Salad with Citrus Sauce

EASY • DO AHEAD   *Serves: 6*

1 small mango, peeled and diced

1 cup fresh blueberries

1 banana, peeled and sliced

1 cup strawberries, hulled and
    cut in half

1 cup red or green seedless
    grapes

1 apricot, seeded and sliced

1 kiwifruit, peeled and sliced

2 tablespoons plus 2 teaspoons
    orange juice

1 tablespoon lemon juice

2 teaspoons honey

⅛ teaspoon cinnamon

Dash of nutmeg

Combine the fruit in a large bowl and mix lightly. Combine the remaining ingredients and mix until blended. Cover and refrigerate the fruit and the sauce until ready to serve. Just before serving, pour the sauce over the fruit and toss lightly.

Nutrition per serving: Calories 92 • Fat 0.5g • Carbohydrates 23g • Protein 1g •
   Cholesterol 0mg • Dietary fiber 3g • Sodium 4mg

Exchanges: 1½ fruit

Carb Choices: 2

Mangoes provide a rich dose of vitamins, minerals, antioxidants, and fiber in a low-calorie, low-sodium package.

Orange-Berry Walnut Cupcakes

EASY • DO AHEAD • FREEZE   *Serves: 24*

1 cup whole-wheat flour
1 cup all-purpose flour
⅓ cup sugar
⅓ cup brown sugar
1½ teaspoons baking powder
½ teaspoon baking soda
¾ teaspoon cinnamon
¾ cup orange juice

¼ cup nonfat vanilla yogurt
¼ cup egg substitute
2 teaspoons grated orange peel
1 cup Craisins
2 tablespoons chopped walnuts
½ cup powdered sugar
2 teaspoons water

Preheat the oven to 350 degrees. Spray two 12-cup muffin pans with nonfat cooking spray. Combine the whole-wheat flour, all-purpose flour, sugar, brown sugar, baking powder, baking soda, and cinnamon in a large bowl; mix well. Combine the orange juice, yogurt, and egg substitute in a medium bowl; mix with an electric mixer (or process in food processor) until creamy and smooth. Gradually add the yogurt mixture to the flour mixture, stirring just until moistened and blended. Fold in the orange peel, Craisins, and walnuts. Fill the muffin cups ¾ full; bake for 20 to 25 minutes, until cooked through. Cool in the pan for 5 to 10 minutes. Remove from the pan and completely cool on wire rack. Combine the powdered sugar and water in a small bowl; mix well. Drizzle the icing over the cooled cupcakes. Let stand for 15 minutes before serving or packaging for storage.

Nutrition per serving: Calories 91 • Fat 0.5g • Carbohydrates 21g • Protein 2g • Cholesterol 0mg • Dietary fiber 1g • Sodium 48mg
Exchanges: 1½ other carb
Carb Choices: 1

Researchers at the University of Western Ontario say that orange juice provides much more than a daily dose of vitamin C—packed with substances that boost good cholesterol, orange juice is considered a heart-healthy beverage.

Raisin Rice Pudding

EASY • DO AHEAD   *Serves: 4*

6 cups water
1½ teaspoons cinnamon
1 cup long- or short-grain rice,
    uncooked

1½ cups skim milk
1½ cups nonfat half-and-half
⅔ cup sugar
¼ cup raisins

Combine the water and cinnamon in a medium saucepan; bring to a boil over high heat. Stir in the rice; reduce heat to low. Cook for 25 to 30 minutes, until the liquid has been absorbed. Remove the pan from the heat; add the milk, half-and-half, and sugar. Cook over medium heat, stirring constantly, until the mixture thickens. Fold in the raisins. Rice pudding can be served hot or cold.

Nutrition per serving: Calories 410 • Fat 0.5g • Carbohydrates 93g • Protein 7g •
   Cholesterol 2mg • Dietary fiber 1g • Sodium 51mg
Exchanges: 6 other carb
Carb Choices: 6

> Short-grain rice, used most often for Asian cooking, contains more amy-lopectin (type of starch) than long- or medium-grain rice, making it more sticky and creamy when cooked.

Sweet Potato Pudding

EASY   *Serves:* 6

1 cup canned sweet potatoes,   ¼ cup **Craisins or dried**
   mashed   **cranberries**
2 bananas, peeled and mashed   1 tablespoon sugar
1 cup evaporated skim milk   1½ teaspoons ground cinnamon
⅓ cup egg substitute   Dash of nutmeg
3 tablespoons brown sugar

Preheat the oven to 325 degrees. Spray a shallow baking dish with cooking spray. Combine the potatoes and bananas in a medium bowl; add the milk, egg substitute, and brown sugar. Mix until completely blended smooth. Spoon the potato mixture into the baking dish. Combine the Craisins, sugar, cinnamon, and nutmeg; sprinkle over the potato mixture. Bake the pudding for 40 to 45 minutes, until a knife inserted in the center comes out clean.

Nutrition per serving: Calories 169 • Fat 0.3g • Carbohydrates 37g • Protein 6g •
  Cholesterol 2mg • Dietary fiber 2g • Sodium 123mg
Exchanges: 2 other carb
Carb Choices: 2

> Yams in the United States are actually sweet potatoes with relatively moist texture and orange flesh. Although the terms are generally used interchangeably, the U.S. Department of Agriculture requires that the label "yam" always be accompanied by "sweet potato."

Upside-Down Ginger-Peach Cake

AVERAGE · DO AHEAD   *Serves: 16*

24-ounce can peach halves,
  canned in juice
1½ cups plus 3 tablespoons
  brown sugar, divided
1½ tablespoons lemon juice
⅓ cup Craisins
1½ cups cinnamon applesauce
3 egg whites, lightly beaten
1½ cups all-purpose flour

1 cup whole-wheat flour
2½ teaspoons baking soda
1 teaspoon ground ginger
1½ teaspoons ground cinnamon
¼ teaspoon nutmeg
¼ teaspoon ground cloves
½ cup nonfat frozen yogurt or 2
  tablespoons nonfat Cool Whip,
  optional

Preheat the oven to 325 degrees. Spray a 9x13-inch baking dish with cooking spray. Drain peaches, reserving 2 tablespoons of juice. Cut the peach halves in half again. Combine the reserved peach juice, 3 tablespoons of the brown sugar, and lemon juice in a small bowl; mix well. Arrange the peaches in the bottom of the baking dish; sprinkle with the Craisins and drizzle with the peach sauce. Combine the remaining ingredients in a large bowl and mix until blended. Pour the batter over the peaches and bake for 35 to 40 minutes, until a toothpick inserted in the center comes out clean. Cool for 5 to 10 minutes; loosen the sides with a knife and invert the cake onto a serving platter. Serve warm with frozen yogurt or Cool Whip, if desired.

Nutrition per serving: Calories 204 · Fat 0.3g · Carbohydrates 49g · Protein 3g · Cholesterol 0mg · Dietary fiber 2g · Sodium 149mg
Exchanges: 3 other carb
Carb Choices: 3

Peaches spoil quickly, so buy just what you need. Look for firm-fleshed peaches without bruises; avoid those with green areas as they were picked too early and will never be as sweet as you'd like. Store hard, unripe peaches at room temperature until soft; ripe peaches should be stored in a plastic bag in the refrigerator, where they will keep for up to five days.

Zucchini Cake with Pineapple and Raisins

EASY • DO AHEAD   *Serves: 16*

½ cup skim milk
1 cup quick-cooking oatmeal,
   uncooked
1 cup crushed pineapple in juice,
   undrained
¼ cup applesauce
2 egg whites, lightly beaten
¼ cup egg substitute
1 teaspoon vanilla

½ cup sugar
½ cup brown sugar
1½ cups whole-wheat flour
1 cup all-purpose flour
1 tablespoon baking powder
½ teaspoon baking soda
1½ teaspoons cinnamon
¾ cup shredded zucchini
½ cup raisins

Preheat the oven to 350 degrees. Spray a 9x13-inch baking dish with cooking spray. Combine the milk and oatmeal in a large bowl; mix well and let stand for 10 minutes. Add the pineapple with juice, applesauce, egg whites, egg substitute, vanilla, sugar, and brown sugar; mix until the ingredients are blended. Combine the whole-wheat flour, all-purpose flour, baking powder, baking soda, and cinnamon in a zip-top bag; shake until the ingredients are blended. Add the dry ingredients to the moist all at once; mix until the ingredients are moistened. Fold in the zucchini and raisins. Spread the batter in the baking dish; bake for 40 to 45 minutes, until a toothpick inserted in the center comes out clean.

Nutrition per serving: Calories 270 • Fat 1g • Carbohydrates 61g • Protein 7g • Cholesterol 0mg • Dietary fiber 4g • Sodium 164mg
Exchanges: 4 other carb
Carb Choices: 4

For best taste, choose smaller zucchini with firm, glossy skin; store them unwrapped in the produce drawer of the refrigerator. To retain maximum vitamins and fiber, do not peel zucchini.

Appendix A

Dr. Edward B. Diethrich and Jyl Steinback Answer Your Questions About *Fill Up to Slim Down*

I thought carbs were the worst thing you could eat if you want to lose weight. Why is *Fill Up to Slim Down* pushing carbohydrates?

Dr. Diethrich: We're not "pushing" carbs with this book. Instead, we're recommending a practical way of eating that will keep you very satisfied, well-nourished, and heart-healthy. If you eat a diet that satisfies you and at the same time protects your heart from coronary artery disease, isn't that a win-win situation, something we should all strive for? Sure, you can eat a diet that eliminates or severely limits carbs, but if it's full of saturated fats and high in cholesterol, the long-term effect on your health is a source of real concern.

But do we really need carbohydrates?

Dr. D: You must eat carbohydrates. To run properly, your body needs a certain amount of sugar. But you don't have to get your sugar allotment from refined sugars found in so many commercial products on the market today. Instead, eat more complex carbohydrates and foods that are sweet in their natural state. What foods are these? Fresh fruits and vegetables, for a start. Whole-grain breads and cereals will also change to sugar in your body, so eat more of them, too. But go easy on table sugar, honey, jelly, candy, and other refined sugar products.

Jyl Steinback: And we're not the only ones who are saying this now. The September 2003 issue of *More* magazine interviewed Dr. Miriam Nelson, author of *Strong Women Stay Slim,* about the impact of diet on building muscle. She commented that following the Atkins diet in the short term may promote rapid weight loss, improving your fat-to-lean ratio in the process. But she added that the benefit comes at "too high a price." If you reduce carbohydrates (in the form of whole grains, fruits, and vegetables), as his diet suggests, Nelson believes that you will be "deprived of key phytochemicals that protect against type 2 diabetes, blindness, osteoporosis, and heart disease." Her recommendations mirror ours: a diet high in fruits, vegetables, and whole grains, with small amounts of protein and fats from healthy sources such as olive oil and nuts.

Both Dr. Atkins and Dr. Agatston, who wrote *The South Beach Diet,* are cardiologists, but their diets limit carbohydrates. They also recommend more fat and protein than the Fill Up to Slim Down plan. Why do doctors who are similarly trained advocate such different programs?

Dr. D: There are many different diets used for weight loss, but none of these programs are based on more than thirty years of research on clinical patients as I have done at the Arizona Heart Institute. While most of these diets have produced short-term weight loss and in some cases, more enduring weight maintenance, most dieters using these and other plans haven't succeeded in achieving long-term healthy weight. What's worse is that they've often sacrificed good health habits for the promise of easy weight loss. For some Atkins dieters, that's meant eating a lot of saturated fat and protein products that may be high in additives. Studies have shown that these foods aren't good for maintaining heart health, especially over a lifetime. My program is based on three decades and thousands of patients, and the foods I recommend promise to satisfy hunger without playing roulette with your health.

I'm worried about how I'm going to like these new foods. And will I really feel satisfied?

Jyl: The food plan in *Fill Up to Slim Down* is designed around foods that make you feel full and help maintain a healthy heart. You'll be eating foods high in soluble fiber, which is great for controlling cholesterol—carrots, barley, legumes (all those tasty beans), rolled oats, and rice and oat bran. A true heart-smart diet includes plenty of whole-grain cereals, brown rice, fruit with peel, and beans (pinto, kidney, navy), and other legumes (black-eyed peas, split peas, lentils). You also want to include substantial amounts of insoluble fiber, found mostly in vegetables, unrefined wheat, and most grains. This kind of fiber speeds foods through your intestinal tract, keeps you regular (*Dr. D:* what we physicians call "increasing fecal bulk"), and delays digestion and absorption of carbohydrates.

I can never figure out what to make for dinner that doesn't take tons of time. What's going to happen when I give up the ease of frozen dinners?

Jyl: They don't call me "America's Healthiest Mom" for nothing! I've provided you with 120 delicious recipes plus a month of mix-and-match menus to help you make great eating choices every day. You'll breakfast on scrumptious baked goods and luscious smoothies, you'll lunch on hearty soups and tasty pasta dishes, you'll dine on delectable fish, chicken, and beef recipes, and you'll enjoy all kinds of great variations on that heart-healthy classic, the potato. Best of all, you'll learn how to incorporate some previously unfamiliar foods into your everyday menus, and I bet they'll soon become family favorites. And if you're a popcorn lover, prepare to enjoy your preferred snack as often as you like.

Think of it this way: *Fill Up to Slim Down* will let you give your family the greatest gift of all: good health that lasts a lifetime. When you all begin to "eat to your heart's desire," you'll quickly feel and look your best ever!

I've been told that I need to avoid foods that are high on the glycemic index, foods like potatoes and carrots. Now you're saying that I can have them again?

Dr. D: While it's true that some individuals experience an increase in blood glucose from eating certain foods, vegetables such as potatoes and carrots are much less likely to cause this problem because they are complex carbohydrates. The health and satiety benefits from eating these high-fiber foods have been proven again and again, so do give them another chance. Once you begin eating for the satiety, you may see much less of a reaction when you consume them as part of an overall program.

I lost weight very fast when I followed the Atkins program, but it came back very quickly when I went off it. What's my chance of keeping the weight off this time around?

Jyl: There's no magic to any diet program—sorry! The Fill Up to Slim Down plan is a real commitment that can work wonders for you. But if you stop doing what works, you're just as likely to see your weight creep up again. So—don't do that! This is a terrific way to nourish yourself and your family, and while it may seem a little challenging at first to eat less protein than you're used to, you may be surprised at how quickly you adapt to the Fill Up to Slim Down program. You know what they say: If you want to see a change, you have to make a change.

Everywhere I look, somebody is coming out with a new low-carbohydrate product. Why is everyone jumping on the bandwagon?

Jyl: I think it's that quick-fix mentality, the idea that right around the corner is the perfect date, the better car, the ritzier home—and the diet that doesn't require any effort. Just remember that all the products you see are making lots of money for their manufacturers. Many of these products vary only slightly from the original versions, but the companies are charging twice or three times as much for the trendy, low-carb repackaging. I say, let the buyer beware!

Dr. D: I just wanted to add that in a recent study published in the *Archives of Internal Medicine*, and widely reported in the popular press, research showed that a high-carb, low-fat diet still delivers reliable weight loss over time. I liked the way reporter Sid Kircheimer described it on WebMD: "How's this for a great way to lose nearly a pound a week: Don't exercise. Don't count calories. Eat until you're full, and oh, yeah, what you eat mostly comes from the newest four-letter word in the dieter's dictionary—'carb.'" This study, which took place at the University of Arkansas nutrition and metabolism lab, noted that even older, overweight people who were diagnosed with pre-diabetes could still enjoy plenty of complex carbohydrates, eat as much as they wanted, and lose pounds. The deciding factor appeared to be keeping fat calories under 20 percent of the total consumed. (Sound familiar?)

Jyl: And don't forget that *USA Weekend* editor Jean Carper actively rebutted the low-carb fad in her column, offering great reasons for continuing to eat your complex carbs. She reported a study from Greece that showed that heart disease risk plunged 72 percent in men and women who ate more than five fruits and vegetables a day, as compared with those who ate less than one a day. She also noted a Vanderbilt University report that said women who ate the most dark yellow-orange and green vegetables had 20 to 35 percent lower odds of breast cancer. Even in Japan, research demonstrated that eating fruits and vegetables every day reduced deaths from liver, stomach, and lung cancer by 20 to 35 percent. Thanks, Jean, for keeping us up to date on such good news!

We understand that you may find it hard to contemplate this new way of eating and living, especially if you've tried many times and then returned to old habits and your old weight. But when you think about what you really want to accomplish, we hope you'll find the courage you need to begin. Wake up tomorrow prepared to move in the right direction, which is ONWARD—Overcome Negativity With A Renewed Desire!

Appendix B

A Month of Mix-and-Match
Menus for Women and Men

Women's Menu

Day	Calories	Breakfast	Lunch	Dinner
Day 1	1,111	Banana Pancakes ½ cup fruit juice of choice	Caesar Crab Salad Rye Crisp crackers	Pan-fried Mahimahi with Horseradish Sauce Balsamic Glazed Portobello Mushrooms ½ cup angel hair pasta
Day 2	1,211	Breakfast Burrito 1 cup cut-up fruit water and lemon	Chef's Ranch Salad ½ whole-wheat bagel	Romaine Salad with low-fat salad dressing Grilled Halibut with Orange Salsa Spinach Risotto
Day 3	1,121	Eggs-traordinary Omelette Florentine 1 slice rye toast with jelly ½ cup orange juice	Fiberful Ranch Salad whole-grain crackers with 2 ounces low-fat cheese Peachy Summer Soup	Lemon Chicken Stir-fry Chinese vegetables Bread stick
Day 4	1,158	Nutty Fruit Salad Cheese and egg-white omelette (made with 4 egg whites and 1 ounce nonfat cheese) 1 cup skim milk	Tarragon Shrimp Salad whole-grain roll Fruit Fantasia	Grilled Chicken Breasts with Papaya Salsa Steamed Asparagus and Peas with Brown Rice

Day	Calories	Breakfast	Lunch	Dinner
Day 5	1,072	Spinach Frittata ½ cup pineapple/orange juice	Tortilla Roll-up with Black Beans baked chips with salsa	Lemon Grouper Soyfully Rich Couscous Spinach Baked Au Gratin
Day 6	1,076	Eggs-traordinary Western Omelette 1 cup strawberries or cantaloupe 1 cup skim milk	Potato-Squash Soup fat-free croutons 1 cup grapes	Salmon Loaf with Dijon Sauce Roasted Vegetables 1 slice garlic bread
Day 7	1,214	Banana Nut Bread Smoothie (blend ½ cup skim milk, ½ cup vanilla yogurt, and ½ cup favorite fresh or frozen fruit with ½ cup ice)	Sweet and Sour Bean Salad Melba or rye crackers with 2 oz low-fat cheese	Italian Lentil Loaf Caesar Salad 1 slice French bread
Day 8	1,124	Eggs-traordinary Mexican Omelette 1 slice rye toast with jelly	Pita Stuffed with Spinach Salad 1 cup fresh fruit	Lemon Cod Apricot-Raisin Noodle Kugel ½ cup green beans
Day 9	1,182	French Toast Pockets ½ cup fruit juice	Honey-Dijon Pasta Salad with Tuna whole-wheat crackers	Bountiful Burger 1 potato (sliced and baked in oven with garlic seasoning) Dinner Salad with low-fat Ranch salad dressing

Women's Menu

Day	Calories	Breakfast	Lunch	Dinner
Day 10	1,102	½ cup whole-grain cereal skim milk ½ banana, sliced	Nutty Fruit Salad French bread roll with 1 tbsp. low-fat peanut butter	Bean and Cheese Burrito baked chips with salsa
Day 11	1,107	Pumpkin Spice Oatmeal ½ cup apple or grape juice	Tarragon Potato Salad Baked Salmon Patties	Main Meal Meat Loaf Baked potato with fat-free sour cream Corn on the Cob
Day 12	1,213	Turkey Vegetable Quiche ½ cup fruit juice	Maestro Minestrone Fat-free croutons + ½ oz Parmesan cheese, shredded, over soup garden salad with low-fat dressing	Crusted Baked Salmon Parmesan Pasta Pilaf Glazed Oranges
Day 13	1,076	Fruit 'n' Yogurt with Kashi ½ cup fruit juice	Fish Chowder in Sourdough Bread Bowl Spinach Salad with low-fat dressing	Lahvosh Vegetarian Pizza Fruit Salad with citrus sauce

Day	Cal.	Breakfast	Lunch	Dinner
Day 14	1,196	2 slices whole-wheat toast with peanut butter; ½ cup strawberries	Very Veggie Stuffed Potato; Chunky Cinnamon Applesauce	Stir-fried Chinese Chicken; ½ cup brown rice
Day 15	1,159	Pumpkin Raisin Muffin; 2 Egg Beater omelette with 1 slice fat-free Swiss cheese	Chicken Vegetable Pasta Salad; 1 slice pita bread	Vegetable Lasagna; Dinner Salad; whole-wheat pita
Day 16	1,152	Berry Breakfast with Crunch Topping	Quick Cream of Broccoli Soup; Sesame Potato Stix	Linguine with Scallops; ½ cup green beans
Day 17	1,090	½ whole wheat bagel, toasted; ½ cup nonfat cottage cheese mixed with 2 tbsp. raisins + 2 tsp. cinnamon; ½ cup apple juice	Chicken and Rice Tortilla Soup; Baked Chips	Simple Seafood Bake; Couscous with Feta and Mint; Garden Salad
Day 18	1,155	Breakfast Muffins with Almond Glaze; Chocolate milk shake (¾ cup skim milk + 1 tbsp. cocoa + ½ cup nonfat vanilla yogurt + ½ banana + 1 tbsp. honey)	Spicy Romaine Shrimp Salad; 1 slice crusty bread; Sweet Potato Pudding	Vegetarian Chili with Beans; whole-wheat crackers
Day 19	1,148	Egg and Tortilla Casserole; ½ cup juice	Wonderful Waldorf Salad; 1 slice bread with 1 oz cheese, melted	Stuffed Sole; Curried Vegetables; ½ cup cooked brown rice

Women's Menu

Day	Calories	Breakfast	Lunch	Dinner
Day 20	1,179	Yogurt Parfait (8 oz nonfat yogurt + 1 cup berries + 1 tbsp. low-fat granola or sliced almonds)	Honey Dijon Pasta Salad with Tuna whole-wheat roll	Turkey Cheese Burgers Fajita-Topped Potatoes
Day 21	1,109	½ cup mini shredded wheat or high-fiber cereal of choice ½ cup skim milk ½ banana	Quick-cooking Vegetable Bean and Rice Soup whole-grain crackers	Orange Roughy Provençale Mediterranean Eggplant Pasta
Day 22	1,104	½ cup oatmeal 2 tbsp. raisins (or fruit of choice) 1 cup low-fat chocolate milk	Chicken and Rice Salad Apple slices	Italian Beef Pita Pockets Vegetable Barley
Day 23	1,146	Fruit & Fiber Breakfast ½ cup juice	Superstar Bean Salad ½ cup nonfat cottage cheese whole-grain crackers	Vegetable Beef Skillet Meal whole-grain roll
Day 24	1,093	Garden Frittata ½ cup juice	Curried Lentil Soup crackers	Stuffed Turkey Loaf Skillet Stuffing ½ cup steamed broccoli

Day	Calories	Breakfast	Lunch	Dinner
Day 25	1,071	Fruitful Pineapple Zucchini Bread Fruity Breakfast Shake (½ cup nonfat yogurt + ½ cup skim milk + ½ banana + ½ cup strawberries + ½ cup pineapple chunks + 2 tsp. sugar + 1 tsp. vanilla + ⅔ cup crushed ice)	Sweet Potato Soup bagel chips Romaine salad with low-fat salad dressing	Orange Chicken Spinach Mashed Potatoes Steamed Asparagus
Day 26	1,157	Veggie White Omelette (2 tbsp. chopped scallions + 2 tbsp. chopped tomatoes + 2 tbsp. chopped bell pepper + ½ cup steamed broccoli + 4 egg whites + 1 oz. fat-free cheese) 1 slice whole-wheat bread, toasted 1 cup skim milk	Southwest Stew	Lentil Chili Pita Triangles Chocolate Almond Cake
Day 27	1,108	1 cup cooked Cream of Wheat ¾ cup blueberries or raspberries or blackberries 1 cup skim milk	Chicken Stew garden salad whole-wheat roll	Simple Stir-fried with brown rice ½ cup mandarin oranges Orange Berry Walnut Cupcake

Women's Menu

Day	Calories	Breakfast	Lunch	Dinner
Day 28	1,129	Mushroom & Broccoli Frittata ½ cup juice Pineapple Orange Muffin	Heart-Healthy Stuffed Cabbage Orzo Pilaf with Artichokes ½ cup raw baby carrots	Lentil Pasta with Diced Tomatoes 1 slice garlic bread Melon slices
Day 29	1,183	½ cup Quaker Multi-Grain Oatmeal + 1 tbsp. brown sugar + ½ banana + ¼ cup skim milk	Pineapple Chicken Packet ½ cup yolk-free egg noodles	Dill Salmon with Vegetables Mango Chutney Rice
Day 30	1,216	Huevos Mexicano 1 cup of cut-up fruit	Chicken and bean tostadas Spanish rice	Cod fillets with Dijon sauce Poppy Seed Coleslaw Orange Sweet Potatoes

Men's Menu

Day	Calories	Breakfast	Lunch	Dinner
Day 1	1,466	Banana Pancakes with 2 tbsp. syrup 1 cup fruit juice of choice 2 slices Canadian bacon	Caesar Crab Salad 2 slices rye bread	Pan-fried Mahimahi with Horseradish Sauce Balsamic Glazed Portobello Mushrooms 1 cup angel hair pasta
Day 2	1,461	Breakfast Burrito 2 slices wheat toast with 2 tsp. jam 1 cup cut-up fruit water and lemon	Chef's Ranch Salad whole-wheat bagel	Romaine Salad with low-fat salad dressing Grilled Halibut with Orange Salsa Spinach Risotto
Day 3	1,462	Eggs-traordinary Omelette Florentine 2 slices rye toast with jelly 1 cup orange juice	Fiberful Ranch Salad whole-grain crackers with 2 oz low-fat cheese Peachy Summer Soup	Lemon Chicken Stir-fry Chinese vegetables 2 breadsticks 1 cup skim milk

Men's Menu

Day	Calories	Breakfast	Lunch	Dinner
Day 4	1,439	Nutty Fruit Salad cheese and egg-white omelette (made with 4 egg whites and 1 oz nonfat cheese) 1 cup skim milk	Tarragon Shrimp Salad 2 whole-grain rolls Fruit Fantasia	Grilled Chicken Breasts with Papaya Salsa Steamed Asparagus and Peas with Brown Rice dinner salad with low-fat dressing and croutons
Day 5	1,445	Spinach Frittata 1 cup pineapple/orange juice 1 cup Simply Potatoes hashbrowns	Tortilla Roll-up with Black Beans 1 cup corn (Mexican-style) baked chips with salsa	Lemon Grouper Soyfully Rich Couscous Spinach Baked Au Gratin
Day 6	1,429	Eggs-traordinary Western Omelette 2 slices whole-wheat toast with jelly 1 cup strawberries or cantaloupe 1 cup skim milk	Potato-Squash Soup whole-wheat crackers 1 cup grapes side salad with low-fat dressing and croutons	Salmon Loaf with Dijon Sauce Roasted Vegetables 2 slices garlic bread

Day	Calories	Breakfast	Lunch	Dinner
Day 7	1,444	Banana Nut Bread Smoothie (blend 1 cup skim milk, 1 cup vanilla yogurt, and 1 cup favorite fresh or frozen fruit with 1 cup ice)	Sweet and Sour Bean Salad Melba or rye crackers with 2 oz low-fat cheese	Italian Lentil Loaf Caesar Salad 1 slice French bread
Day 8	1,509	Eggs-traordinary Mexican Omelette 2 slices rye toast with jelly 1 cup fruit juice	Pita Stuffed with Spinach Salad 1 cup fresh fruit 1 cup low-fat cottage cheese	Lemon Cod Apricot-Raisin Noodle Kugel ½ cup green beans
Day 9	1,482	French Toast Pockets 1 cup fruit juice 1 cup lowfat yogurt	Honey-Dijon Pasta Salad with Tuna 2 wheat rolls	Bountiful Burger 1 potato (sliced and baked in oven with garlic seasoning) Dinner Salad with low-fat ranch salad dressing
Day 10	1,427	1 cup whole-grain cereal skim milk 1 banana, sliced	Nutty Fruit Salad 2 French bread rolls with 2 tbsp. low-fat peanut butter	Bean and Cheese Burrito baked chips with salsa
Day 11	1,417	Pumpkin Spice Oatmeal 1 cup apple or grape juice 1 cup low-fat yogurt	Tarragon Potato Salad Baked Salmon patties Caesar salad with low-fat dressing and croutons	Main Meal Meat Loaf baked potato with fat-free sour cream roasted vegetables

Men's Menu

Day	Calories	Breakfast	Lunch	Dinner
Day 12	1,472	Turkey Vegetable Quiche 1 cup juice Cran-Apricot Oatmeal Bar	Maestro Minestrone Fat-free croutons + 1 oz Parmesan cheese shredded over soup Garden salad with low-fat dressing	Crusted Baked Salmon Parmesan Pasta Pilaf Glazed oranges
Day 13	1,546	Fruit 'n' Yogurt with Kashi 1 cup fruit juice	Fish Chowder in Sour-dough Bread Bowl Spinach Salad with low-fat dressing	Lahvosh Vegetarian Pizza Fruit Salad with citrus sauce Raisin Rice Pudding
Day 14	1,455	2 slices whole-wheat toast with peanut butter 1 cup strawberries 1 cup skim milk	Very Veggie Stuffed Potato Chunky Cinnamon Apple-sauce	Stir-fried Chinese Chicken 1 cup brown rice
Day 15	1,504	2 Pumpkin Raisin Muffins 2 Egg Beater omelette with 1 slice fat-free Swiss cheese 1 cup fruit juice	Chicken Vegetable Pasta Salad 1 slice pita bread	Vegetable Lasagna dinner salad with low-fat dressing 2 whole-wheat rolls

Day	Calories	Breakfast	Lunch	Dinner
Day 16	1,424	Berry Breakfast with Crunch Topping 1 cup low-fat yogurt 1 cup fruit juice	Quick Cream of Broccoli Soup Sesame Potato Stix	Linguine with Scallops ½ cup green beans
Day 17	1,418	1 whole-wheat bagel, toasted 1 cup nonfat cottage cheese mixed with 2 tbsp. raisins + 2 tsp. cinnamon 1 cup apple juice	Chicken and Rice Tortilla Soup baked chips	Simple Seafood Bake Couscous with Feta and Mint garden salad
Day 18	1,406	2 muffins with almond glaze Chocolate milk shake (¾ cup skim milk + 1 tbsp. cocoa + ½ cup nonfat vanilla yogurt + ½ banana + 1 tbsp. honey)	Spicy Romaine Shrimp Salad 2 slices crusty bread Sweet Potato Pudding	Vegetarian Chili with Beans whole-wheat crackers 1 cup fresh fruit
Day 19	1,447	Egg and Tortilla Casserole ½ cup juice 2 slices Canadian bacon	Wonderful Waldorf Salad 2 slices of bread with 2 oz cheese, melted	Stuffed Sole Curried Vegetables 1 cup cooked brown rice
Day 20	1,529	Yogurt Parfait (8 oz nonfat yogurt + 1 cup berries + 1 tbsp. low-fat granola or sliced almonds) 1 whole-wheat bagel with 2 tbsp. low-fat peanut butter	Honey Dijon Pasta Salad with Tuna whole-wheat roll	Turkey Cheeseburgers Fajita-Topped Potatoes

Men's Menu

Day	Calories	Breakfast	Lunch	Dinner
Day 21	1,423	1 cup mini shredded wheat or high-fiber cereal of choice 1 cup skim milk 1 banana	Quick-cooking Vegetable Bean and Rice Soup whole-grain crackers	Orange Roughy Provençale Mediterranean Eggplant Pasta
Day 22	1,472	1 cup oatmeal 2 tbsp. raisins (or fruit of choice) 1 cup low-fat chocolate milk	Chicken and Rice Salad apple slices 2 whole-wheat rolls	Italian Beef Pita Pockets Vegetable Barley
Day 23	1,443	Fruit & Fiber Breakfast 1 cup fruit juice	Superstar Bean Salad ½ cup non-fat cottage cheese whole-grain crackers	Vegetable Beef Skillet Meal whole-grain roll
Day 24	1,468	Garden Frittata 1 cup fruit juice 3 vegetarian bacon strips	Curried Lentil Soup crackers salad with low-fat dressing, croutons, and 1 oz low-fat cheese	Stuffed Turkey Loaf Skillet Stuffing ½ cup steamed broccoli 1 cup skim milk

Day	Calories	Breakfast	Lunch	Dinner
Day 25	1,432	Fruitful Pineapple Zucchini Bread Fruity Breakfast Shake (1 cup nonfat yogurt + 1 cup skim milk + 1 banana + 1 cup strawberries + 1 cup pineapple chunks + 4 tsp. sugar + 1 tsp. vanilla + ⅔ cup crushed ice)	Sweet Potato Soup bagel chips Romaine salad with low-fat salad dressing and croutons	Orange Chicken Spinach Mashed Potatoes Steamed Asparagus 1 cup skim milk
Day 26	1,455	Veggie White Omelette (2 tbsp. chopped scallions + 2 tbsp. chopped tomatoes + 2 tbsp. chopped bell pepper + ½ cup steamed broccoli + 4 egg whites + 1 oz. fat-free cheese) 2 slices of whole-wheat bread, toasted 1 cup skim milk	Southwest Stew 2 pieces garlic toast 1 cup grapes	Lentil Chili Pita Triangles Cinnamon-Spiced Baked Banana
Day 27	1,429	1 cup cooked Cream of Wheat ¾ cup blueberries or raspberries or blackberries 1 cup skim milk	Chicken Stew Garden salad with croutons 2 whole-wheat rolls	Simply Stir-fried with Brown Rice 1 cup mandarin oranges 2 Orange Berry Walnut Cupcakes

Men's Menu

Day	Calories	Breakfast	Lunch	Dinner
Day 28	1,409	Mushroom & Broccoli Frittata 1 cup fruit juice 2 Pineapple Orange Muffin	Heart-Healthy Stuffed Cabbage Orzo Pilaf with Artichokes 1 cup raw baby carrots	Lentil Pasta with Diced Tomatoes 2 pieces garlic bread melon slices
Day 29	1,438	½ cup Quaker Multi-Grain Oatmeal + 1 tbsp. brown sugar + ½ banana + ¼ cup skim milk apple slices	Pineapple Chicken Packet ½ cup yolk-free egg noodles	Dill Salmon with Vegetables Mango Chutney Rice
Day 30	1,439	Huevos Mexicano 1 cup cut-up fruit	Chicken and bean tostadas Spanish rice	Cod fillets with Dijon sauce Poppy Seed Coleslaw Orange Sweet Potatoes

Index